WRITING WITH LIGHT

Photographs by

Robert Merrill Eddy

Meditations and music by

Kathy Wonson Eddy

WRITING WITH LIGHT

meditations for caregivers in word and image

Foreword by Henri J. M. Nouwen

United Church Press
Cleveland, Ohio

United Church Press, Cleveland, Ohio 44115

© 1997 by Robert Merrill Eddy and Kathy Wonson Eddy

Printed in the United States of America on acid-free paper

02 01 00 99 98 97   5 4 3 2 1

Library of Congress Cataloging-in-Publication Data
Eddy, Robert Merrill.
    Writing with light : meditations for caregivers in word and image /
photographs by Robert Merrill Eddy ; meditations and music by Kathy Wonson
Eddy ; foreword by Henri J.M. Nouwen.
        p. cm.
    ISBN 0-8298-1166-4 (pbk. : alk. paper)
    1. Caregivers—Religious life.   2. Helping behavior—Religious aspects—
Christianity—Meditations.   I. Eddy, Kathy Wonson, 1951– .   II. Title.
BV4910.9.E33 1997   96-51907
242—dc21   CIP

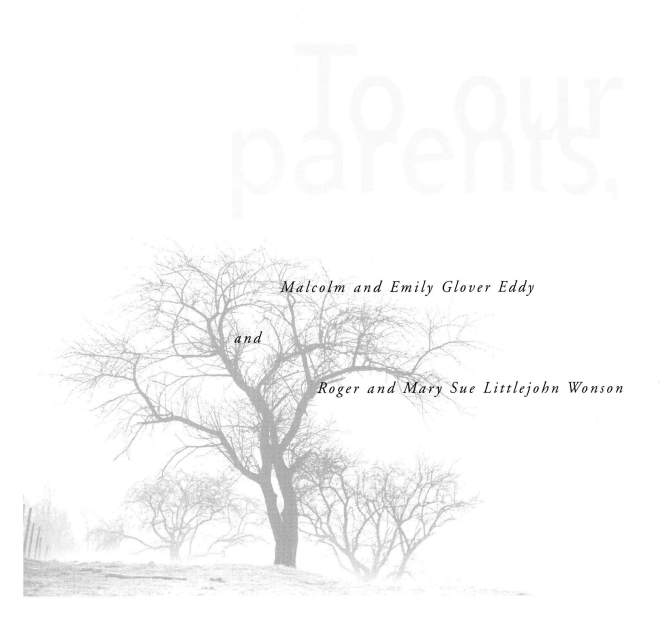

To our parents,

Malcolm and Emily Glover Eddy

and

Roger and Mary Sue Littlejohn Wonson

Foreword

To care is to be truly present to the moment and discover right there the presence of God. This beautiful book for caregivers shows this care through word and image.

Each photograph and meditation makes you stop, think, and wonder, and leads you deeper into the heart of God. A mother kissing her child, the radiant face of a young woman, a little boy looking at a spider's web, two teenagers imitating the picture of a dancer, an elderly couple holding hands, a young woman looking in a mirror, one teen touching gently the belly of another pregnant teen, a man listening attentively to two children, the grateful face of a Jamaican man, a mechanic climbing under the hood of a car, a long lace dress moving in the wind—it is life, it is love, it is prayer, it is human, it is divine.

Robert Merrill Eddy's evocative photographs and Kathy Wonson Eddy's penetrating observations tell us more about caregiving than many books on pastoral theology because they call us to be fully present to the moment and fully trust that God is here and now.

So often we think or speak about the life of contemplation as the opposite of the life of action. But this book reveals that they belong together, yes, that they are the two aspects of care. Contemplation is sensing God in the moment. Action is helping

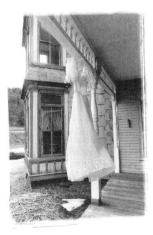

others sense God in the moment. Caregiving is giving eyes to see and ears to hear the movements of God's Spirit right where we are.

Paul writes to the Corinthians: "The Spirit searches everything, even the depths of God. . . . No one comprehends what is truly God's except the Spirit of God. Now we have received not the spirit of the world, but the Spirit that is from God, so that we may understand the gifts bestowed on us by God" (1 Corinthians 2:10–12).

This splendid book is a truly spiritual book because it looks at the day-to-day—seemingly so ordinary—events with the eyes of God and reveals there the unfathomable mystery of which we are part. It sees and makes us see and thus searches the depths of God in creation.

When I looked at the photographs and read this book, I was struck by the choice facing us. We can choose to see just misery and failure, pain and conflict, anguish and agony, but we can also choose to see, in the midst of all the darkness that surrounds us, the light of God's face. A caregiver is one who always chooses the light.

Bob and Kathy have given all caregivers—and who is not a caregiver?—a very precious gift, indeed a gift written in the light. I hope and pray that all those who take this book in their hands, open it, look at its photographs, and read its words will shout with joy, "My soul proclaims the greatness of my God."

Henri J. M. Nouwen

who

Words of Introduction from the Photographer

The word "photography" comes from the Greek words meaning "to write with light." Most of the images in this collection were gathered in my work as photographer for *The Herald of Randolph,* a small weekly newspaper serving several towns in central Vermont.

Each week I go out into the world to chronicle moments of significance on the emulsion inside my camera. This is a mysterious process, for it fuses that which is happening "out there" with my own vision. The latent image lies on the boundary of the camera's film plane, a space between the photographer and the event. This space is profoundly sacred. While I am out in communi-

is not a caregiver?

ty "gathering light," I confess I am not always aware of this. But there are many moments while composing an image in the lens of my eye that I am surprised by that which is Wholly Other. The moment seems lit by meaning more than by light.

Sometimes it seems that this significance can be reflected on the film. Perhaps this is where photography begins.

The gathering of the images in community is the journey outward. This is balanced at *The Herald* by a journey inward. In the small space of the darkroom, with the white noise of running water and air shutting out the sounds of office and street, the film's images are written with light onto the surfaces of sensitive paper. The printing process is essentially a dance as my hands move over the surface of the print, blocking and permitting light to shine in greater and lesser degrees on parts of the image needing to be brought up or down.

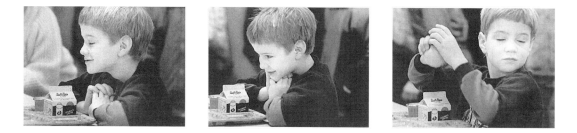

The result? These are honest attempts to be present to that moment of original encounter when I, camera in hand, glimpsed something sacred and sought to convey its meaning to others.

Once, when a breakfast program was beginning in a local elementary school, I photographed a young boy savoring an orange in his mind and then attempting to peel it. The images of that encounter remind me that the holy is all around and within us. May we each have eyes to see.

Robert Merrill Eddy

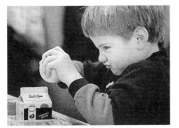

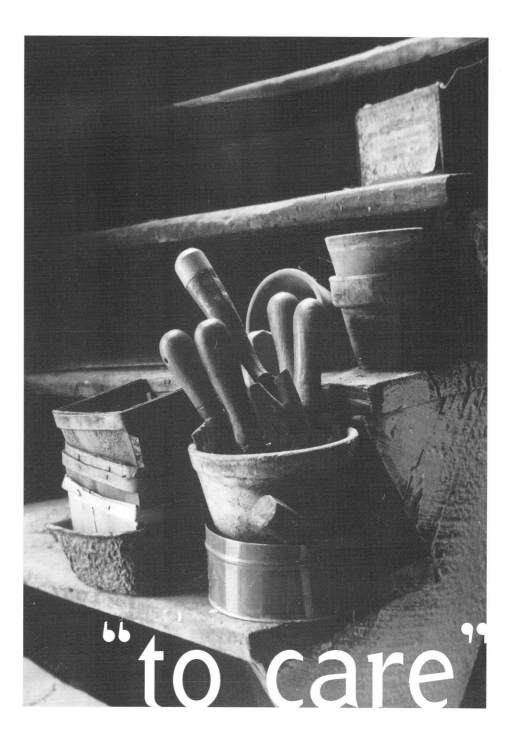

"to care"

Words of Introduction from the Author

I have been a pastor of a three hundred-member UCC church in central Vermont for twenty years. I was surprised early in my ministry to learn how many people do not realize the value of their caring; most are unaware of the profound significance of their loving words and actions in another's life. Rabbi Abraham Heschel's words, "Know that every deed counts, that every word is power," are needed urgently as this century closes (see p. 83). Our caregiving is important in the universe.

The Indo-European root of "to care" is *gar,* to "cry or call." Closely related are ancient words in English and German for sorrow, grief, and lament. Thus the earliest meaning for "to care" involved simply being with persons in their sorrow, hearing their cry, helping them give voice to their lament. There is an element of "enoughness" in these early language roots that we have lost. We need to learn again that our presence is enough. It is enough just to be with someone, to offer ourselves, to give our full attention. It is a great gift to "rejoice with those who rejoice, weep with those who weep" (Romans 12:15).

Who are caregivers? Nurses, ministers, social workers, doctors, teachers of preschoolers through post-doctoral students, hospice volunteers, people who work in nursing homes, twelve-step group members, church committee members, church school teachers, funeral directors, volunteers in schools and hospitals, therapists, and parish visitors are caregivers. Personnel directors in corporations, people who care for the elderly, school secretaries, members of guidance departments, seminary students, medical technicians, members of Interfaith Caregivers Network, workers in substance abuse centers or health clinics, senior citizen advocates, directors of volunteers in community organizations, inner-city grassroots workers, and daycare providers are caregivers. Nurses' aides, people who clean or cook for others, ambulance and emergency room workers, and all who care for those who are mentally ill or physically challenged are caregivers. Yet the term "caregivers" applies to more than those whose professional lives are in the service arena. All parents, grandparents, spouses, and friends, anyone who cares for another in love, is a caregiver. *Writing with Light* is for us all.

Burnout is high in caregiving. This book encourages an in-depth relationship with God, who is the source of all our energy for service. Sabbath time taken each day refreshes us, renew-

for

ing our minds and bodies in the never-ending wellspring of God's shalom. Time apart for play and prayer teaches us to look at others (and ourselves) with eyes of love. In the midst of responsibility we find ourselves surprised by peace and joy; our daily tasks are transformed into shining occasions of grace. What was burdensome becomes an opportunity for service with a light heart.

As you gaze at these photographs, sing these songs, and reflect on these meditations, may you discern the light-filled writing of God in your own heart. May you discover God's luminous calligraphy in your life each day.

Kathy Wonson Eddy

opportunity service with a light heart.

WRITING WITH LIGHT

Swish.

Hiss.

As the bicycle wheels move through the water a broad wake behind sings, "Someone has passed here! Someone has made a difference!" The boy on the bike is unaware of the wide effect of his passing. He doesn't see the shimmering movement of molecules he has caused, or the beauty of light and shadow on the ridges of water extending from his bike, fluid curves, a water smile.

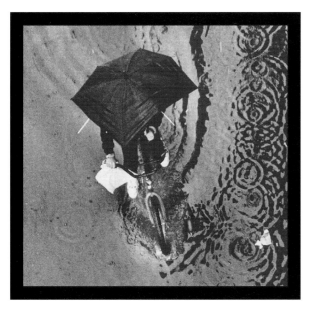

Ping.

Plop.

Rain dripping from the edge of a tenement roof creates a pattern of interwoven circles. Like Venn diagrams superimposed one over another, they dance above the pavement. These watery mandalas call the eye to the center, but there is always movement outward. Nothing is static, nothing is stationary. The water is always moving out from the center to touch other circles one by one. Droplets that fell separately from the roof's edge now are linked through these liquid rings expanding outward. At water's edge the circles become densely packed, and the design resembles phrase markings in music. Curved lines on a musical score indicate that the notes below are to be connected, played smoothly without a break. Here, as the boy with the broken umbrella rides past litter and halos of water and light, the curved phrase lines tell of the graceful legato of God underlying all things. For God, all things are connected, linked, without break or barrier, joined, fastened.

Swish.
Hiss.
   Ping.
Plop.

Such undignified words!

Pieces of trash littering the watery street: so unsightly!

When we care for others, the work can be undignified and messy. Often we know not the value of the care we give. We do not see the loveliness in our wake, the grace in another's life created by our small acts of love. The service we offer leaves a wide and beautiful design.

It is our center in God that gives us the impetus and energy to reach out and link with others. Always from that center we flow outward. The center first, then the reaching out. The center first.

Rain drips from a tenement roof and a pattern of exquisite beauty emerges, intersecting circles moving outward, connecting, connecting, connecting. Simply putting our arms around another begins a growing circle of love whose broad reaches are beyond our imaginings. We offer a touch, a word, a gesture, and change in the world begins.

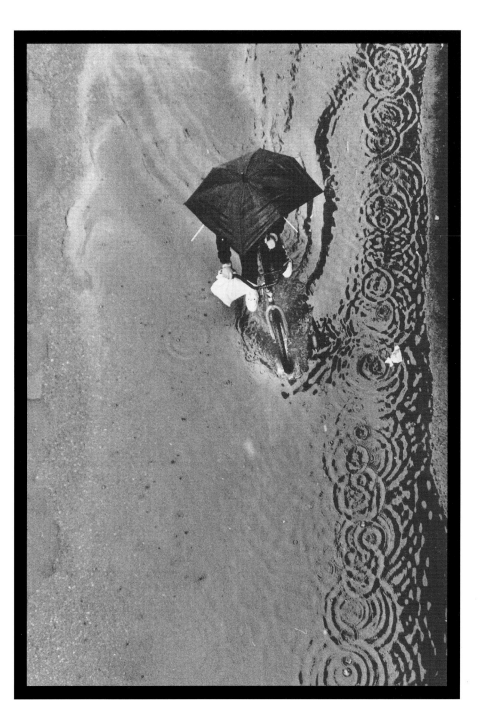

We offer a

touch, a word,

a gesture, and

change in the

world begins.

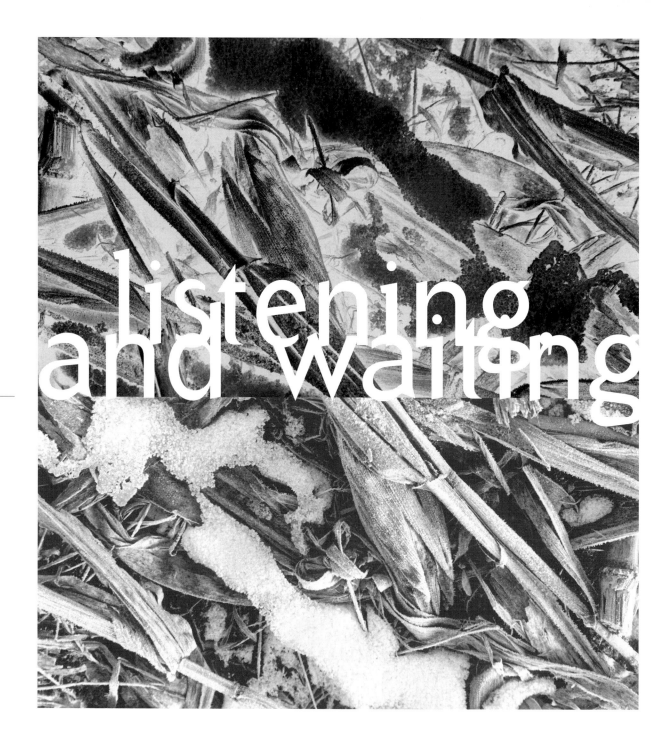

listening
and waiting

In the season of late fall, the cloudy sky is gray and lifeless, almost pressing on our shoulders. For many people this is a time of dread. Even those of us who enjoy skiing alpine fields or tramping in snowy woods anticipate the coming of winter with anxiety and reluctance. We fear driving on treacherous icy roads and the growing isolation and restlessness. We resent the annoyance of salty puddles on our floors from snow-laden boots and the endless shoveling and plowing, dressing and undressing children. Winter's approach colors November days.

And yet it is precisely when we are burdened with winter-fear that the November cornfield cries out, "Come and see. Look! Gaze with openness and love. I will teach you of the Now."

Intently examine the cornfield at left. Do you see the grasses lacing up a cornhusk shoe, the bow tie of looped husk strips, the needles of frost pricking the air? See! The frost stitches the edges of leaf and stalk to the chilled sky. Sparkling embroidery is on every surface. Beauty emerges as we gaze. There is quietness in these stalks: their work is done. The frenzy of growth and fruitfulness, summer's breakneck pace of cell division and multiplication, is over. Peace is here. Now in your imagination lift your eyes from the ground to gaze at November trees lining the borders of the cornfield, all leaves stripped away, bare branches sewing the gray clouds to the land, a ravelled seam at the horizon. When we turn our thoughts away from fear of winter's coming to gaze around us, we see the beauty of the Present, crystalline and sparse.

In our caregiving, when dread of some future difficulty or pain overtakes us, it is time to stop. Stop. Breathe deeply in and out. See the beauty emerge close at hand. God says, "I am here, now, in this moment. Be in this moment, quiet and still. I give you myself, and that is all you need." Fallow time for looking, listening, and waiting enriches us the way the soil of earth's fields is nourished in the long deep quiet between harvest and planting. When we take this time, our fears for the future—"Can I face what lies ahead? Will I have the energy and skill to offer the care required of me?"—become as evanescent as frost that disappears at the touch of a warm fingertip.

The Now is endlessly mystical and transforming. When we stop and gaze we are astounded to discover at the edges of our fears the jewelled stitchery from God's hand, the embroidery of Love sewing our days together in all seasons.

Today,
look at the world
with eyes of peace.

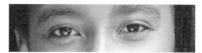

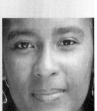

with

eyes of peace.

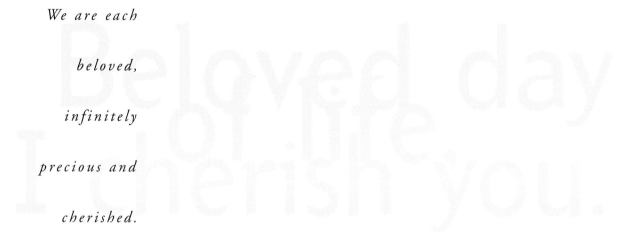

We are each

beloved,

infinitely

precious and

cherished.

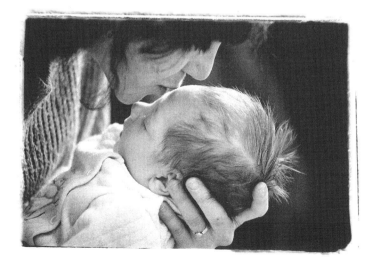

The mother and the light kiss the baby's forehead. The child is utterly relaxed and trusting in its mother's arms. Held securely from beneath, blessed with warm breath and delicate touch from above, the child simply receives. Love is poured out and nothing is required in return. Even so God holds us. We are each beloved, infinitely precious and cherished. We can rest deeply in God, bathed in light, confident in the strong and tender arms that support us. We can be at peace. What a profound difference is made in our caregiving when we are truly conscious throughout the day: "I am held by God!" Free from the need to impress others, to be above reproach, to act out of guilt or fear, to rush to meet tight schedules, we carry the peaceful knowledge within that God sustains us in all things. God's breath—*ruach, pneuma,* the Holy Spirit—lightly brushes the face of our minutes and days as a sign of how much we are loved. Psalm 131 sings of God holding us:

> But I have calmed and quieted my soul
> Like a child quieted at its mother's breast;
> Like a child that is quieted is my soul.
> —*Psalm 131:1–2 (RSV)*

Yet there is also another way to live out the truth of this image. Yes, we are the child loved tenderly by God, but we can be the mother also. Think of this day, today, as something of immeasurable value and worth that you have been given. Hold this day of your life tenderly. Love this day. With gentleness greet it with a light kiss. Hold it dear. Whatever demands this day might make of you, savor it as the gift it is.

Beloved day of life, I cherish you.

The spider is a creature of mystery to many Native Americans, and it often has a benevolent and potent role in their legends. Peter Wakefield experienced an encounter with Mystery when he discovered this orb weaver spider's web in the West Brookfield church. See the brilliant light on this delicate sphere of glistening silken threads, a luminous orb shining. Notice the light everywhere: lining the rungs of the upturned chair, resting on the pew's curved wooden arm touched by centuries of hands, dancing on new leaves visible through the ancient wavy glass. Elongated rectangles of light grace the back of the pew and softer light illumines the hand-planed wainscoting. The Mystery is not just in the glowing web, but everywhere! Perhaps this is part of the mystery that Native Americans know the spider to proclaim.

Spiders have much to teach caregivers. Extraordinarily adaptable, spiders can be found in tropical jungles, on polar ice, at the 22,000-foot height of Mount Everest. Adaptability is significant in caregiving, whether we are engaged in teaching, ministry, medicine, volunteering, parenting, caring for the elderly or dying, or listening to another's pain. When we let go of rigidity and our need for predictability, the care we give glistens with light.

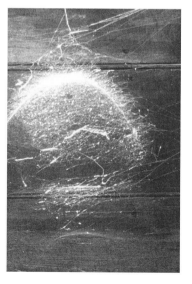
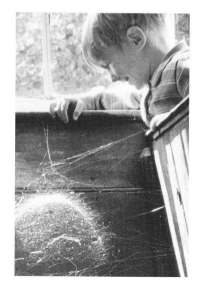
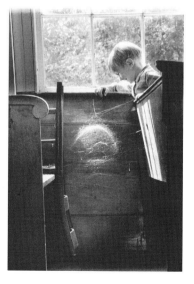

The spinning of an intricate web involves an unbelievable number of repetitions. Back and forth. Back and forth. We can't count the number of large attachment threads in this photograph, much less the tiny threads woven into the sphere. Much of our caregiving, too, is comprised of repetitive tasks. It is easy to become weary and resentful. Over and over we wash off the top of the high chair, dispense medicine and explanations, listen to the same problems, volunteer the same service countless times. The spider teaches us that all this repetition has a purpose, and is even beautiful. Look again at the photograph: the place where the light glows brightest is where the silk is densest, where the most repetition has taken place. New depths and patterns are created with each pass over the same area. All our repeated tasks are opportunities for God's light to grow in us.

Receive the orb weaver's blessing: may you weave the qualities of adaptability and repetition without resentment into the light-filled web of your work.

Remember: spiders spin their silk out of their own bodies. We also have everything we need to provide loving service. Everything we require lies within us. All things necessary are already ours. Herein lies the Mystery.

repetition

Because truly, when people think that they are acquiring
more of God in inwardness, in devotion, in sweetness,
and in various approaches than they do by the fireside
or in the stable, you are acting just as if you took God
and muffled God's head up in a cloak and pushed God
under a bench!

—*Meister Eckhart (1260–1327)*

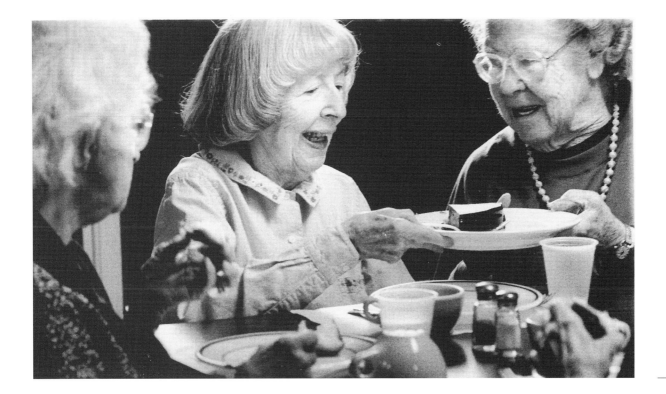

sweetness

Meister Eckhart, Sermon 5b, "In hoc apparuit charitas dei in nobis," in
Meister Eckhart, Classics of Western Spirituality series, translation and
introduction by Edmund Colledge and Bernard McGinn (New York:
Paulist Press, 1981), 183. © 1981 by Paulist Press. Used by permission.

We Want to Love

Words: Brian Wren, 1985, 1994   Music: Kathy Wonson Eddy, 1995

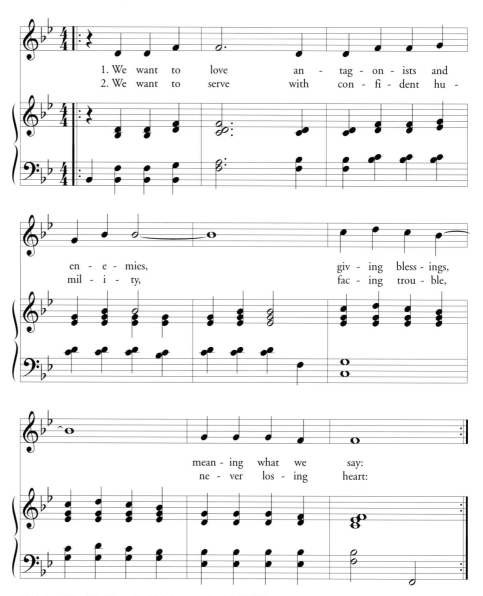

14

1. We want to love an-tag-on-ists and en-e-mies, giv-ing bless-ings, mean-ing what we say:
2. We want to serve with con-fi-dent hu-mil-i-ty, fac-ing trou-ble, ne-ver los-ing heart:

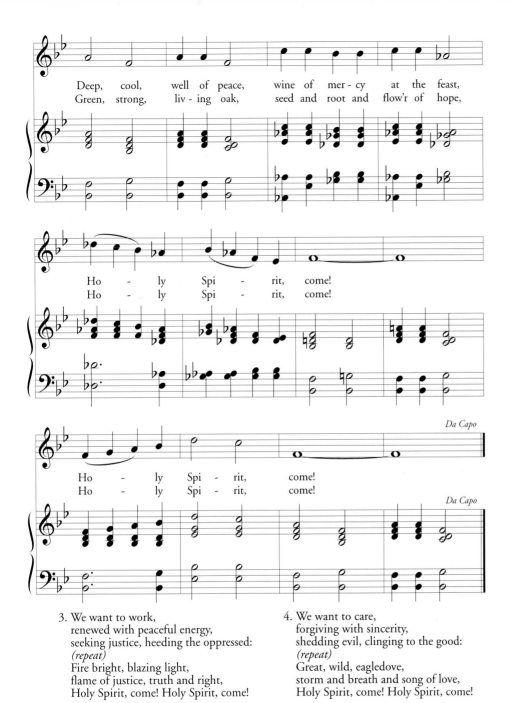

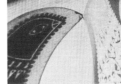

Deep, cool, well of peace, wine of mer-cy at the feast,
Green, strong, liv-ing oak, seed and root and flow'r of hope,

Ho — ly Spi — rit, come!
Ho — ly Spi — rit, come!

Da Capo

Ho — ly Spi — rit, come!
Ho — ly Spi — rit, come!

Da Capo

15

3. We want to work,
   renewed with peaceful energy,
   seeking justice, heeding the oppressed:
   (repeat)
   Fire bright, blazing light,
   flame of justice, truth and right,
   Holy Spirit, come! Holy Spirit, come!

4. We want to care,
   forgiving with sincerity,
   shedding evil, clinging to the good:
   (repeat)
   Great, wild, eagledove,
   storm and breath and song of love,
   Holy Spirit, come! Holy Spirit, come!

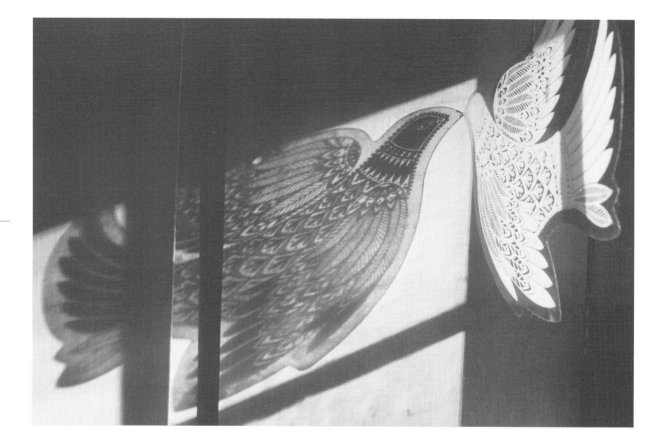

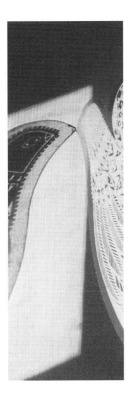

"We Want to Love" was composed for the 1996 New England Pastors Study
Conference, Springfield, Massachusetts. Each verse can be sung by a
soloist and then repeated by the congregation, or the first time
through by the men, then the women, with everyone together on the
last two lines each time. This is especially effective when danced by a
liturgical dancer as the soloists sing each verse.

Sometimes I see images when I pray. I quiet my mind and in the silence pictures float up; they often bring a feeling of catharsis and healing. One August when I was feeling discouraged about ministry and my creative life, I decided to bring the depression to Jesus and then simply wait quietly and watch to see what Christ would do. To my surprise Jesus took a broom and began sweeping me off!

"What are you sweeping off?" I asked.

Jesus answered, "All your NOs, all your CAN'Ts."

Then in my mind's eye, Jesus sprayed me with refreshing water from a hose. The water was filled with the word "Yes" printed in different sizes and styles. The Yes words stuck all over me. Later that day in meditation with a Catholic priest with whom we met weekly for prayer, I "saw" the Yes words in my lungs. With every breath they bounced around and danced. The image made me smile then, and even now as I write of it.

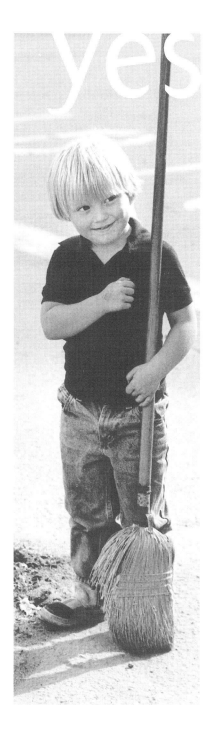

Sweeping removes what is old and clears the way for what is new; it can help us find what was lost. Jesus used a woman sweeping as a metaphor for God:

> Or what woman having ten silver coins, if she loses one of them, does not light a lamp, sweep the house, and search carefully until she finds it? When she has found it, she calls together her friends and neighbors, saying, "Rejoice with me, for I have found the coin that I had lost." Just so, I tell you, there is joy in the presence of the angels of God over one sinner who repents.
>
> —*Luke 15:8–10*

vigorously

brushing

away all

that clutters

and dims

your shining

light.

Today when you take up a broom, think of God sweeping out your mind and heart, vigorously brushing away all that clutters and dims your shining light. God is clearing and preparing a place for your Yes: Yes to this work, this person, this opportunity for love and service, this Now with all its gifts. Yes is the bright coin found in the dust: you actually had it all along and only temporarily misplaced it. God is sweeping your life. *Yes.*

When working for publication, photographers rarely expect to get more than one or two photographs from a thirty-six-exposure roll of film. It is a given that there will be many tries, many not-quite-acceptable prints; this willingness to risk mistakes is an essential part of the creative process.

At the time the Berlin Wall came down, in late fall 1989, Bob was in a field photographing Christ Church of Bethel, Vermont. A flock of forty or fifty pigeons were roosting on the steeple. From across the valley with a 300mm lens he watched the light on the birds and the two-hundred-year-old wood. Bob discovered that if he clapped his hands the birds would fly up, circle in the air, and then settle again on the steeple. Even with the temperature hovering near zero, standing in snow up to his knees, snow filling his cuffs and short boots, he was fascinated by the play of light on the birds' wings as they floated down to land. Several times he clapped his hands and then set the motor drive to click off a burst of exposures. Later in the darkroom he discovered that out of three-and-a-half rolls of film, only one picture captured all the birds in the frame landing with wings opened and full of light. Out of one hundred and twenty shots, one photograph.

Peacemaking, like photography, often has many failed attempts. Working for peace between individuals or nations involves a willingness to try over and over, to make mistakes, to know that reconciliation is never instant but the fruit of a process with many efforts falling short. Strangely, reconciliation involves clapping as well. When we show our appreciation of someone, barriers are broken apart, hostility begins to melt. Genuine recognition of gifts brings people together. Visible signs of gratitude dismantle the walls created by fear and defensiveness.

We will always associate this photograph with the Berlin Wall coming down, as if the three doves offer a trinity of blessing on the reunification, as if one man's clapping half a world away in a snowy field could help take down the wall and applaud the path to peace.

Peace-making

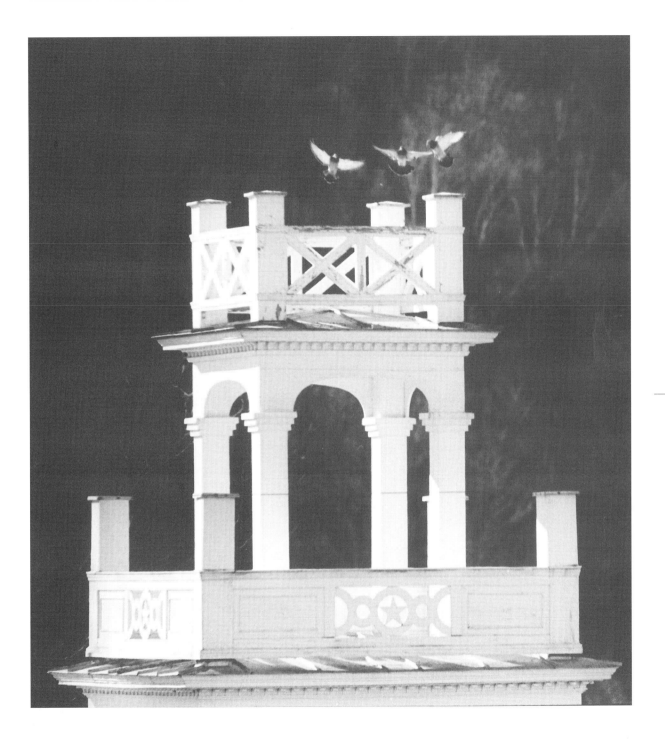

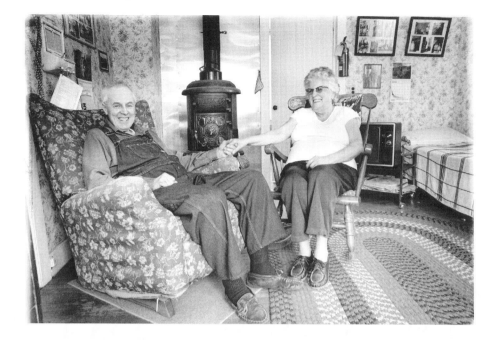

God makes the rivers to flow
They tire not,

    nor do they cease from flowing.

May the river of my life
flow into the sea of Love
that is the Lord.

                        —Prayers from the Rig Veda

f l 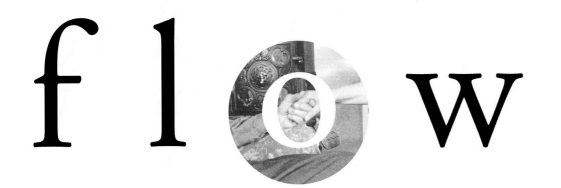 w

This photograph was taken just before a moment of

discovery.

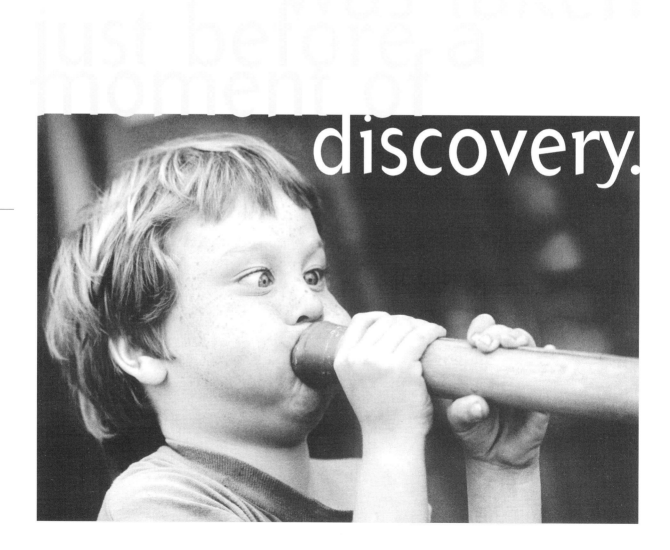

The didgeridoo is an Australian wind instrument played for centuries by the native people from the Outback. Didgeridoos are made from bamboo or from trees hollowed out by insects. They create an eerie sound, a low, breathy moan. At a street fair in Vermont, Bob enjoyed photographing people of all ages trying to make music through this simple instrument.

With puffed cheeks, eyes bulging, and face growing scarlet, Tara strained to make a sound. The harder she blew, the more difficult it became. Then suddenly Tara discovered that if her cheeks and lips were more relaxed, if she didn't try so hard, the haunting, airy notes would come easily. In fact, the only way to create sound was to be at ease.

When Bob told me about Tara as he showed me this photograph, I felt I was being given a lesson from "down under," from the underside of my busy conscious life. In Tara's discovery I heard a call to do ministry in a new way, a way involving less pushing, striving, and accomplishing tasks, and more effortlessness, peace, yielding, and trust. All my life I have chosen the difficult way, equating working hard with my sense of worth. A feeling of being burdened by arduous self-imposed expectations often accompanies my days. There is a wiser path.

I wrote in my journal, "Yahweh, breath of my heart, loving Spirit who forgives all things, wise Teacher who knows the way of yielding, not pushing, I pray for your healing." As often happens (coincidence? synchronicity?!), soon afterward I saw a truck with the bumpersticker "Easy Does It." Easy does "do" it! The peaceful yielding Way is what brings results; the path of simplicity and ease is actually what accomplishes things. The music comes when we give up trying so hard.

Haunting song lines from down under are in Jesus' words:

Come to me, all you that are weary
and are carrying heavy burdens, and I
   will give you rest.
Take my yoke upon you, and learn from
   me
For I am gentle and humble in heart,
And you will find rest for your souls.
For my yoke is easy, my burden is light.
           —Matthew 11:28–30

Once more I had a reminder of the gentler Way.

Florence Scholl Cushman was a soloist with the Chicago Symphony in 1913; the applause after her performance of a Tchaikovsky piano concerto was so prolonged she had to return to center stage for bows eight times. Now 103 years old, Florence lives in Randolph, Vermont, and taught in her studio until just last year. It's a joy to watch her play; her gnarled hands, soft and relaxed, lightly move up and down the keyboard. The touch is so gentle. Ethereal music emerges. I was astonished the first time I went to a recital of her students: they had all learned her light touch, even the youngest beginners. I had expected to hear lots of pounded open-fifths in the left hand, a favorite "pirate" song of early students. Instead one child after another brought beauty and grace to the instrument. It seemed they had absorbed her quietness, and it flowed out of them as fingers lightly brushed the keys.

This day may you bring the light touch to your caregiving: may you choose gentleness with yourself, gentleness with others. Often during the day listen for the soft sounds. See in your mind's eye these time-worn hands, relaxed, yet sure, grazing the keys, moving with peace.

Today, in all you do, the light touch.

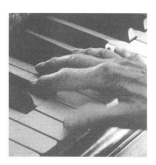

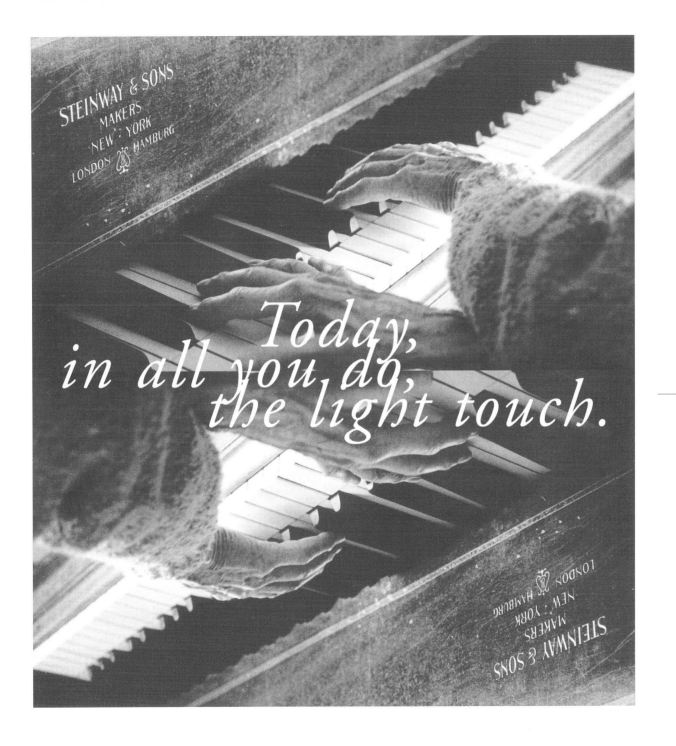

Today, in all you do, the light touch.

Easter Call to Prayer

Words and music: Kathy Wonson Eddy, 1995

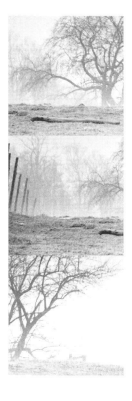

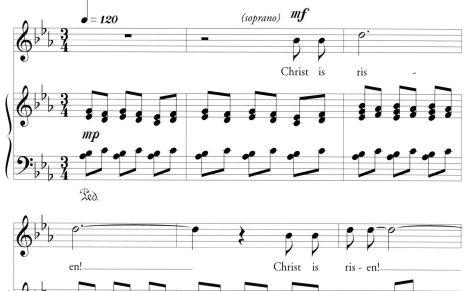

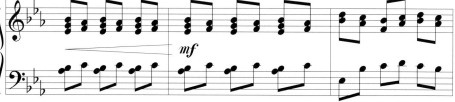

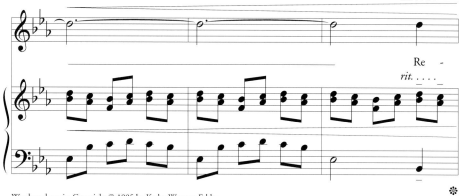

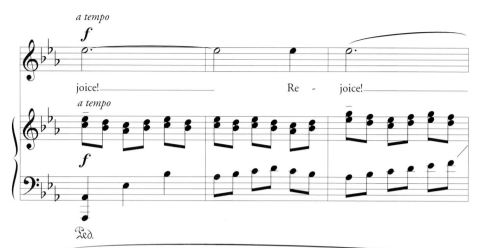

joice!_____ Re - joice!_____

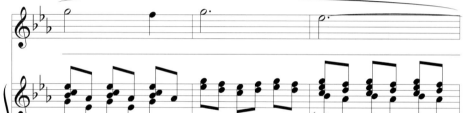

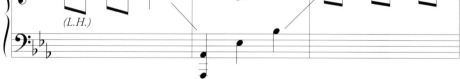

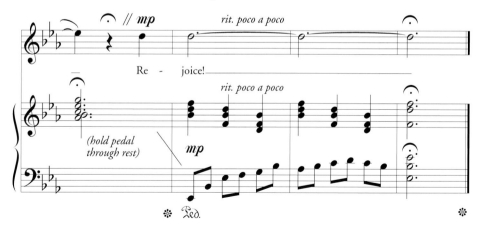

Re - joice!_____

rejoice

For soprano and piano. This can be sung on Easter Day before the prayers of the people. After the liturgist concludes the prayer and before the final amen is spoken, this piece can be repeated by the soprano and piano.

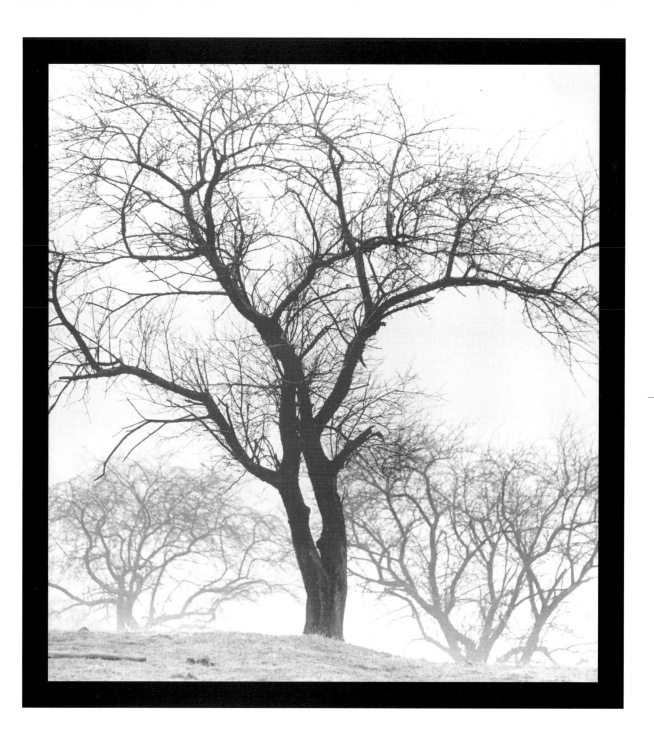

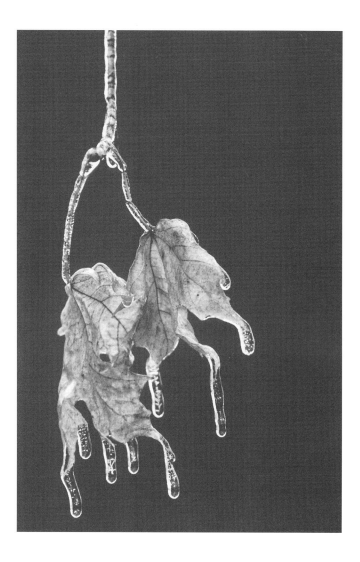

answer

The answer
is always
a form of forgiveness
for ourselves
or for others.

—Lee Colt

Dances

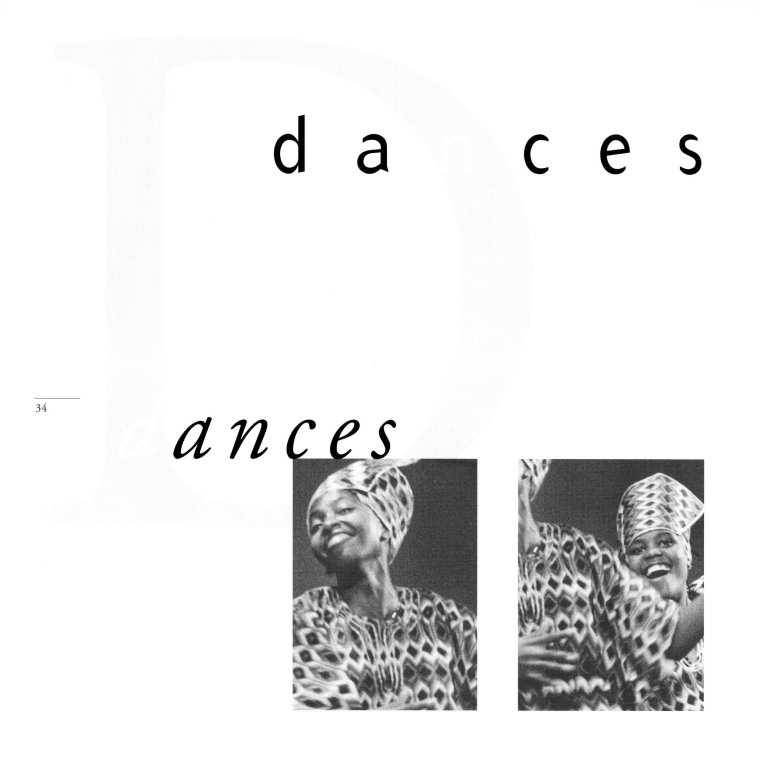

Years ago a parishioner sent us a card we put on our kitchen windowsill to cherish every day. Now faded and stained, it still proclaims in crooked letters, "Joy is the most infallible sign of the presence of God." The truth of these words became evident to our community as South African young people sang their joy and gladness in June 1995 in our town's music hall. God was present, blazing, in their music, drumming, and exuberant movements. The eighteen-voice chorus, Dundee Voices of Joy, from the township of Dundee in South Africa brought Vermonters to their feet clapping and stomping in response to the vibrant music, a spiral of rejoicing and praising God. The Africans in brightly patterned clothes dazzled us with their traditional Zulu songs, rhythms, and dances. Just a year earlier these singers would not have been allowed to leave South Africa because of apartheid. As they sang of freedom their joy was palpable. With arms outstretched, heads flung back, bodies swaying, faces shining, they shared their gladness and delight with

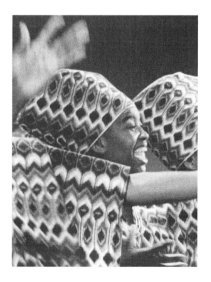

abandon. At the close of the evening the Voices of Dundee and the voices of Vermont stood together to sing the Pan African national anthem in Zulu.

Joy is the most infallible sign of the presence of God. How closely the streams of joy and suffering flow together! The sign of "Jesus" in American Sign Language is a motion that points out the nailprints in Jesus' palms. Thus Jesus is primarily identified as one who suffers. To say Jesus' name in sign language one must recall his physical suffering for the sake of all humanity. These South Africans consider it an inexpressible gift to love a God who knows their pain. And even now, though apartheid is officially over, there is a long road, probably centuries long, to racial equality. Trust in a God who joins them in their trials is what undergirds their music and communal life. For us in the United States who have grown accustomed to freedom and peace, these singers from Africa proclaiming joy out of incredible suffering are agents of God to awaken us.

Our own acquaintance
with grief informs our caregiving.
The pain we have known sensitizes us to
the suffering of others and increases our capac-
ity for compassion and loving service a hundredfold.
When we have known the utterly dependable presence of
God in times of grief and despair, we have an invaluable gift to
offer others. And when we shine forth joy and gladness despite the pain
of life, it is God who dances between us and the people we serve.

With the light touch of finger to palm we proclaim the name of Jesus as one who
is always present when there is suffering. It is our call with gesture and touch to sing other
names for God: the One Who Walks Beside, the Cradler, the Hope-Weaver, the Invincible
Freedom Worker, the One Who Holds Gently, the One of Sorrows Acquainted with Grief, the
Midwife of Joy.

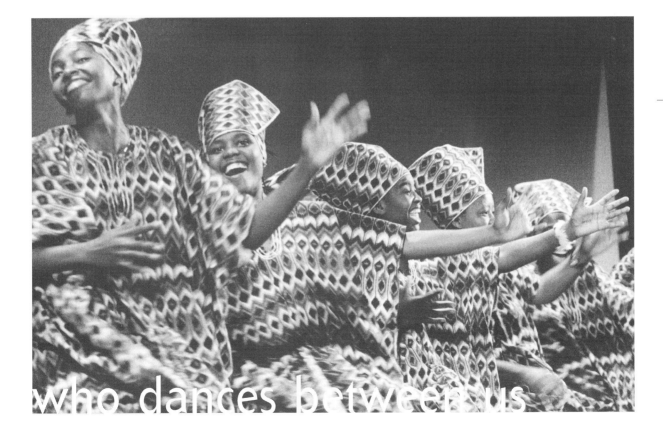

who dances between us

Creating art is a way of serving people. It takes courage and discipline and trust. In February 1994 I felt blocked in composing an anthem that had been commissioned by Pilgrim Church in Duxbury, Massachusetts, to celebrate its 150th anniversary. Every time I sat at the piano to write, the critical part of my mind would judge the notes as trite. I became increasingly afraid as two weeks went by with just truncated jottings on the page. One morning when I prayed about it, I was given an image of angels all around the piano. At noon that day I went to a journaling group meeting at our church where about ten women each week began their time together with silence for journaling. I decided to write a dialogue with the angels, a technique I often use with dream images or in addressing God with questions. I write the questions, and I am always surprised by the ways I am led to answer them. Here is what emerged:

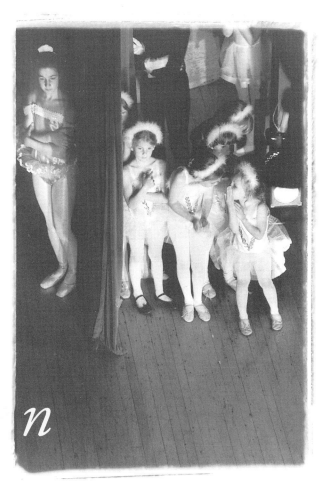

K: Why isn't the music coming?

ANGELS: Because you don't love the little beginnings and trust they will grow into something.

K: What should I do?

ANGELS: Write the small things. That is enough. They will grow.

K: Are these bits of melodies and harmonic ideas okay or should I start over?

ANGELS: Start with them. They are enough for now and they will grow in directions you can't foresee.

K: Why should I be surprised by that prospect? Have I lost hope?

ANGELS: Your judgment is especially strong and critical right now; the judging part of you doesn't trust that newness will come, and bless, and bloom.

K: How can I make the critical voice less strong?

ANGELS: You need more space and time for play. Do not judge your music before it can grow and flower.

K: I've been like this a long time. I need your help. I am afraid, and it feels like creativity is drying up.

ANGELS: We will help you. Inside you we beat our wings and hum. We fill you with love and surround you with love. We are here to help. Open the doors of your mind. Look on us with wonder. Let us sing in you, then write our song. It has already begun. Wait till you hear it! It is beautiful! Listen!

The next morning before composing, I continued this dialogue:

K: Now I go to the piano. I ask your help. I am afraid nothing will come.

ANGELS: Do not fear. Do not take every moment as a test. You have time for nothingness. Out of gestation comes birth.

K: So just keep going to the piano, keep trying?

ANGELS: No, not "trying." Go to the piano to be, to listen. We angels are singing within you. Just listen and you will hear. Write it down. The music of heaven!

O Wind of Heaven, brisk and free,

In us arise,

fill all

our work and prayer.

40

O Wind of Heaven, brisk and free,
In us arise, fill all our work and prayer.
Clothe us in God's tender breath,
A sea of healing air.

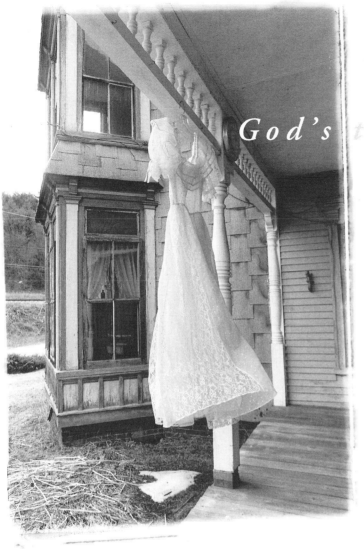

Clothe us in *God's* tender breath,

A sea of healing air.

"O Wind of Heaven, Brisk and Free" (Copyright © 1996 by Kathy Wonson
Eddy) was the text for the first verse of the theme song for the Third
National UCC Women's Meeting in Boston, June 1996.

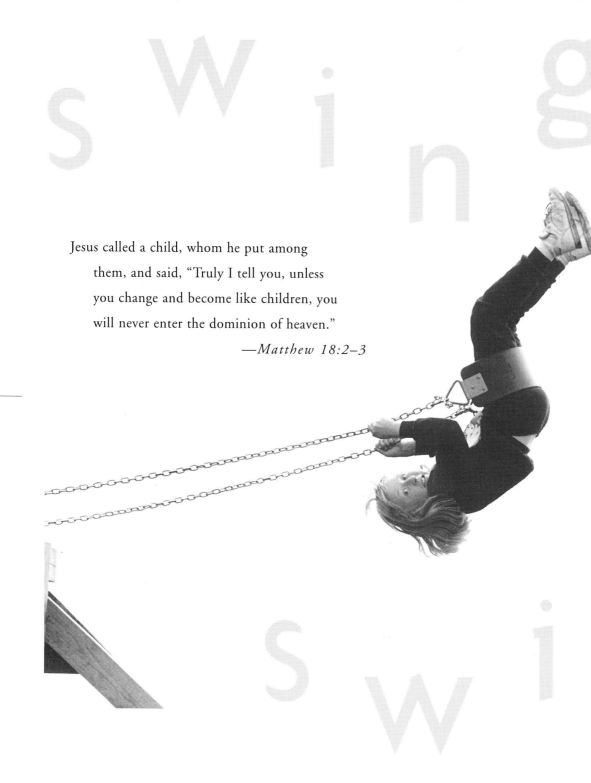

swing

Jesus called a child, whom he put among
them, and said, "Truly I tell you, unless
you change and become like children, you
will never enter the dominion of heaven."
—*Matthew 18:2–3*

"What do I do when my service for others has lost meaning?" a woman asked.

Here are some seeds for new life. Pick one or two:

✔ Swing on a swing set. Pump hard, then float, sail!

✔ Take a walk, watch ants, skip.

✔ Sit by a river and listen.

✔ Vary your daily routine: indulge in sleeping late or get up early to go right outside and let the morning sky greet you.

✔ Do one kind thing for yourself every day. What will it be today?

✔ Gaze at a single flower in a clear glass vase. See the silvery beads on the stem underwater; notice the veins in the petals illuminated by sunlight.

✔ Visit an older person.

✔ Chew gum and smack your lips.

✔ Lie on the ground. In winter make a snow angel; in summer watch clouds and stars.

✔ Clean out a drawer or a pile of clutter; you are also throwing away worn-out ideas about yourself and your work.

✔ Make something with your hands; do not judge your creativity.

✔ Sing.

✔ Plan a trip, even if you don't take it.

✔ Put on loud music and dance to it.

✔ Call up an old friend, someone who thinks you are fantastic, someone who is accepting and forgiving and zesty and laughs a lot. (If you can't think of a soul to call, go back to cleaning out a drawer: throw away the idea that there is no one to call. Someone will pop into your head.)

✔ Take a nap in the sun. This is especially healing in winter: find a place where sun streams through a window into your face. Lie in a patch of sun on the floor.

✔ Smell clean sheets drying on the clothesline.

✔ Think of five things you love to do that you rarely give yourself permission to do. Write them down. Do one of them. Then do another.

Holy Spirit Be at Home in Me

Words and Music: Kathy Wonson Eddy, 1985

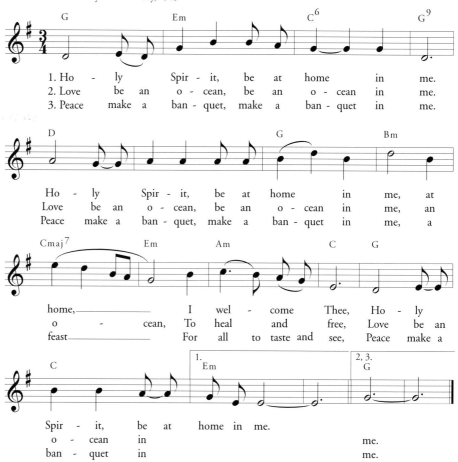

1. Ho - ly Spir - it, be at home in me.
2. Love be an o - cean, be an o - cean in me.
3. Peace make a ban - quet, make a ban - quet in me.

Ho - ly Spir - it, be at home in me, at
Love be an o - cean, be an o - cean in me, an
Peace make a ban - quet, make a ban - quet in me, a

home, I wel - come Thee, Ho - ly
o - cean, To heal and free, Love be an
feast For all to taste and see, Peace make a

Spir - it, be at home in me.
o - cean in me.
ban - quet in me.

be at home in me

This can be sung unaccompanied or with a simple improvised arrangement on available instruments. Cello, piano, baritone horn, violin, and two-part voices have been used at Bethany Church.

44

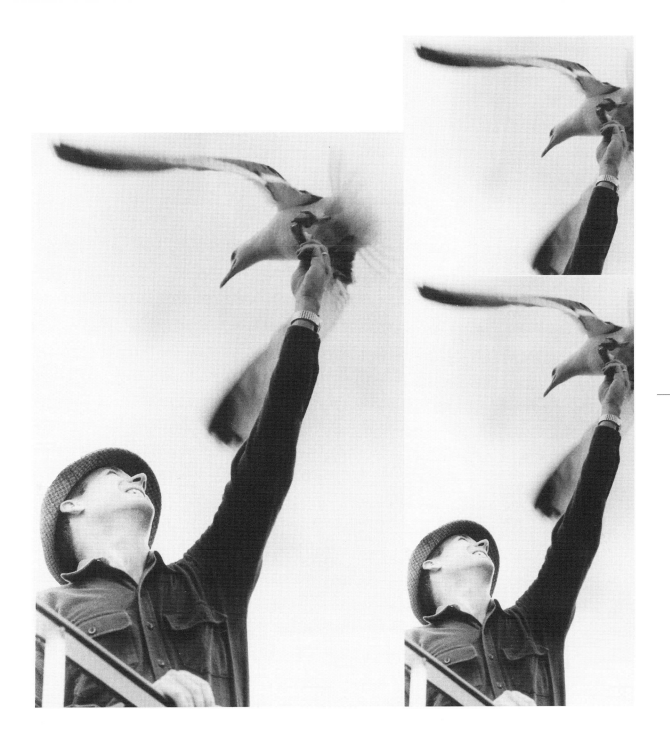

The future of the world
hangs on the breath
of schoolchildren.

—Sayings of the Rabbis,
The Talmud

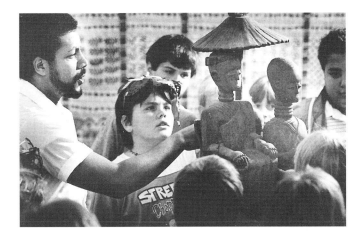

We thank Rabbi Minard Klein of Chicago for sharing this saying of the
Rabbis in the Talmud.

healing

I like knowing

where the

treasures are

within walking

distance of

my home.

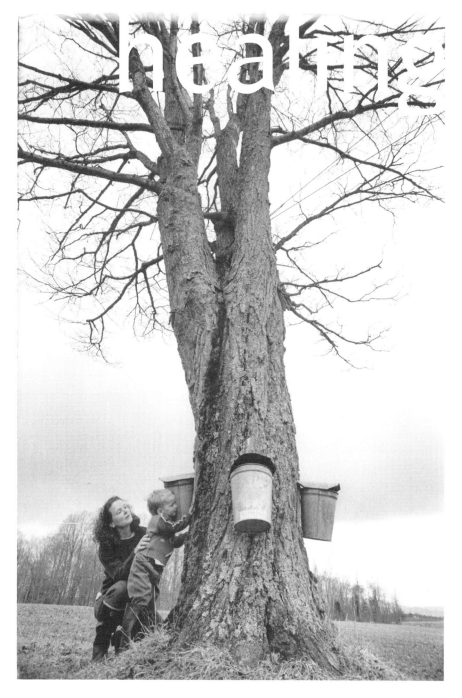

The sap is flowing! It is a treasure in early spring to hear the first plink in the sap bucket, to taste the sweet water.

I like knowing where the treasures are within walking distance of my home. I like knowing where the wild turkeys often feed in the cornfield, where there is lacy pale-green lichen growing on evergreen branches, where in the deep woods you can hear the liquid music of the hermit thrush. I like being aware of the place where there is a profusion of pink lady's slippers, or where suddenly in the woods there is a broad avenue of grass lined by old maples on both sides, a wide roadway of light and airiness. One place I love to visit feels mystical. It is a spring in the forest where among green moss-covered rocks, clear cold water bubbles up from the earth. It is a holy place. Even as I write now, the water is springing up there, always. It is always flowing up, a wellspring.

Inside every person is a well-spring, a *well*-spring, a fountain of wellness, of wholeness, from the Spirit of God. I like to imagine the cool mossy place in my heart, the sun dappling the rocks and wet leaves, the moss emerald and sparkling, the water making soft gurgling sounds and growing, growing to become a rushing stream. The miracle is that this holy wellspring is in everyone else too. How the world would be different if every time we looked at someone, we saw the green place of flowing water within them, the holy spring! This is especially important when there is someone we interact with frequently in our caregiving who irritates us, whose values, mannerisms, or opinions are annoying to us. If you return over and over to the fountain-in-the-woods in your own heart, if you see the wellspring in the other, healing can begin to flow between you. So often what we hate in another is really an

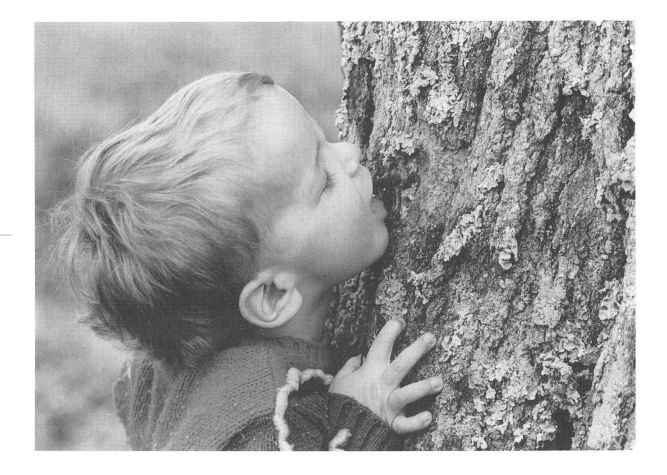

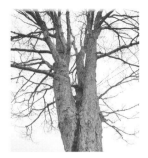

O taste and see

that God is good!

—*Psalm 34:8*

O taste and see

that God is good!

For several weeks I kept this photograph on my sermon desk to ensure I would see it every day. I needed to gaze at it when I felt a lack of focus and energy. Whenever I discerned a need for renewed commitment, this image seemed to say, "Hey! Time to roll up your sleeves and get into it!"

To give our full attention, our energy, our particular gifts, our time brings rich rewards beyond our most extravagant dreams. Our call is to spend our love with delight, not hold it back. It is God who gives us the strength of mind and body to offer ourselves freely. It is God who places in us the renewed desire to care with depth and fullness. The letter to the Ephesians promises that God's "power at work in us is able to accomplish abundantly far more than all we can ask or imagine" (Ephesians 3:20).

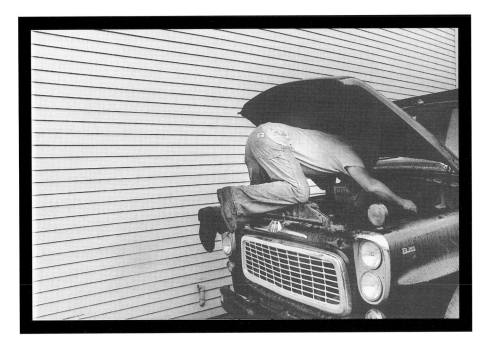

The mechanic's body language communicates that he is offering his best to this task; he is intensely focused and giving all he can. Jesus taught that when we give this way the blessings come flowing back to us:

Give and it will be given to you.
A good measure, pressed down,
Shaken together, running over,
will be put into your lap;
for the measure you give
will be the measure you get back.

—Luke 6:38

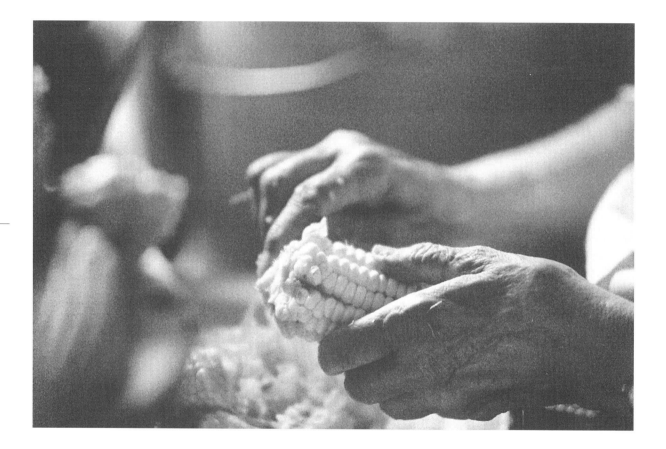

those who
love
those who
labor

One arrangement of this hymn is for the choir or congregation to sing the first verse, the baritone horn to play the melody down one octave (as an interlude verse), then the third verse to be sung with baritone horn countermelody as written.

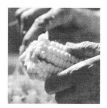

Those Who Love and Those Who Labor

Words: Geoffrey Dearmer (b. 1893), alt.

Music: Kathy Wonson Eddy, 1986

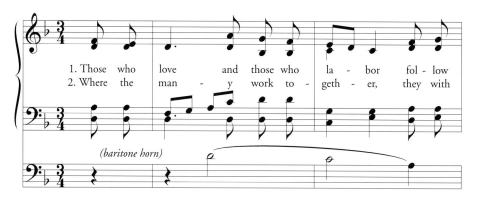

1. Those who love and those who la- bor fol- low
2. Where the man- y work to- geth- er, they with

(baritone horn)

58

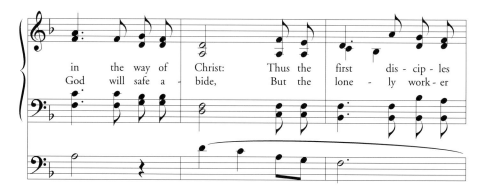

in the way of Christ: Thus the first dis- ci- ples
God will safe a- bide, But the lone- ly work- er

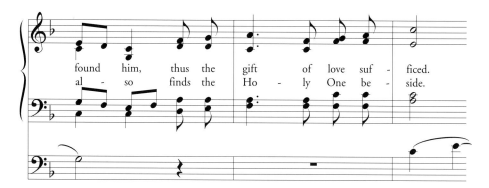

found him, thus the gift of love suf- ficed.
al- so finds the Ho- ly One be- side.

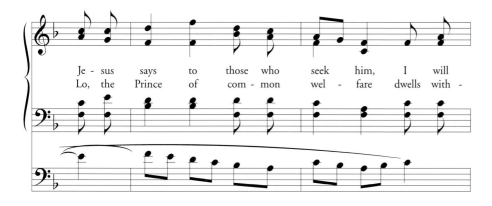

Je - sus says to those who seek him, I will
Lo, the Prince of com - mon wel - fare dwells with -

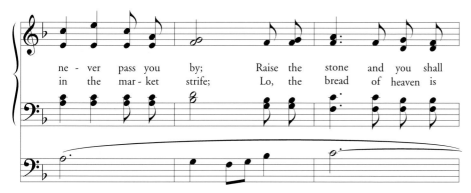

ne - ver pass you by; Raise the stone and you shall
in the mar - ket strife; Lo, the bread of heaven is

59

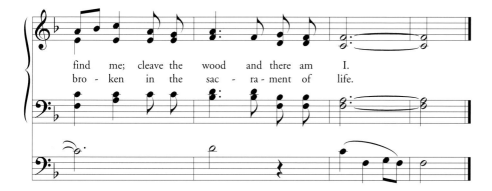

find me; cleave the wood and there am I.
bro - ken in the sac - ra - ment of life.

April Fool's Day comes infrequently on Thursday, the day our local weekly newspaper is printed. The last time it coincided with press day, the staff celebrated with a fake front page replete with outlandish stories and this photograph of a car sunk in mud up to its windows. (Actually, Bob hired an auto body shop to cut the top off of a totaled car and place it in the muddy road. We won't say which town's road because the road crew is still mad at us for printing this picture in the paper, implying that they really do let their roads get this bad.)

Some people say Vermont has only three seasons: winter, the Fourth of July, and mud season. Depending on whom you ask, mud season lasts three weeks to almost three months, with the worst in March and early April. We live about two-and-a-half miles from the nearest paved road, and usually for a few days every mud season we have to leave our car in the village and travel back and forth in our old plow truck with a high carriage. Mud season leads to deep philosophical questions such as, "Why is it that I live here? What could I do to make a living in Fiji or the Sahara?"

In truth, mud season only once a year in the world of nature is a light sentence; mud season of the heart can come at least once a week! We stand, bewildered like the man leaning over his car in the mud, asking, "How did I get myself into this mess?" Entrenched in the quagmire of unhealthy patterns of thinking and acting we realize once again that the only way out is to get help. Through talking to another and listening deeply to our inner life we can be drawn out from the mud of our own making. Slowly we learn how to avoid the sinkholes and ruts, humbled by the knowledge of how easily we get stuck and how much we need a power greater than ours to get us moving again.

Expressions of our need for God to help draw us out of the mud predate tow trucks and Vermont backroads. The nineteenth-century shape note hymn "Wondrous Love" goes, "When I was sinking down, sinking down,

The wonder of it is,

we continually discover that

what we thought

was impassable swamp

is actually the starting place

for a new journey.

journey

sinking down, when I was sinking down, sinking down, when I was sinking down, . . . Christ laid aside his crown for my soul." (Now there's an author not afraid to show how much sinking we can know!) An anonymous Middle English manuscript contains the call to Jesus, "with love cords, draw Thou me." In 1925 Percy Dearmer wrote the beautiful hymn text "Draw Us in the Spirit's Tether." These images of being drawn by God are found in the word "religion" itself. Literally "religion" means to be bound again, relinked, from the Latin word *religare* (*re-*, "back" + *ligare-,* "to fasten, to bind"). Our faith is the living tether, the towrope, the links of chain that fasten us to a God who lovingly draws us to a life of fullness and meaning. Often, though, it is more like being towed than drawn, so great is our resistance to new life, to change and growth! The wonder of it is, we continually discover that what we thought was impassable swamp is actually the starting place for a new journey.

Great journeys always begin in foolishness: foolish dreams, foolish hopes, foolish goals, or so they seem in the eyes of the world. There are plenty of mud holes along the way. Yet as caregivers we are fools of April, the month of rebirth and flowering, all year long. We know mud season won't stop us. If anything, it strengthens us by teaching us again how trustworthy is our God. God the tether-forger, with the very Breath of Heaven, dries the muddy places in the landscape of our hearts. To our astonishment we are once again on firm ground, and we begin a fresh journey, responding to the call to new opportunities for growth and service. With love cords may God draw you; may you know the Spirit's tether of foolishness and joy.

we are once again

on firm ground

God dries the

muddy places

in the

landscape of

our hearts

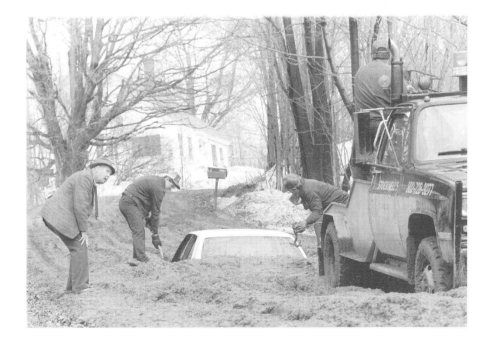

Today
be aware
of God's aboutness.

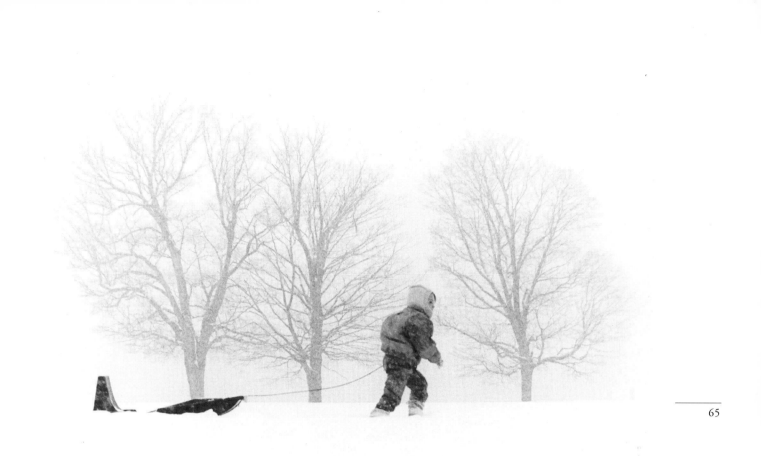

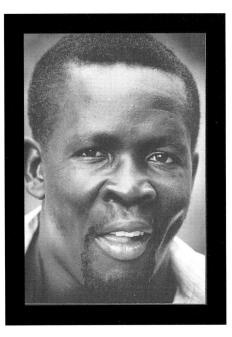

George Simpson came from Jamaica for two summers to work at an organic vegetable farm in Randolph Center, Vermont. He lived in our neighborhood and often came to the parsonage on hot summer evenings to talk and laugh with us on our steps. He said wise and surprising things, and we were aware how much he had to teach us about migrant farmworkers, about poverty, about hope, about God. We invited George to preach at Bethany Church in 1989, and his words challenged our complacency:

In Jamaica, we are poor. Sometimes I wake up in the morning, and there is only tea in the house. I get down on my knees and say, "Thank you, God, for the tea." In America, you have so many things. Yet I am confused: I see so much around me, in your country, but I don't see your people saying, "Thank you, God."

George Simpson, as quoted in *Gifts of Many Cultures: Resources for Worship for the Global Community,* ed. Maren C. Tirabassi and Kathy Wonson Eddy (Cleveland, Ohio: United Church Press, 1995), 13. © 1995 by Maren C. Tirabassi and Kathy Wonson Eddy. Used by permission.

old sorrows

are brought

to light,

and in the

fragrant

summer air

all is made

well.

hearts are stirred

There is nothing in the world as sweet as the smell of new mown hay.

After the hay is mown and lying on the ground, it is stirred up with a tedder. In the morning as soon as the dew is gone the tedder is drawn over the field. It lifts the hay, turning the underlayers up to the drying power of the sun. Fluffing hay up off the ground allows air to circulate, removing moisture before baling. Stirring up the hay with a tedder is not a once-and-for-all process; it may have to be done three or even four times before the hay is dry enough to bale.

In haying, stirring up is a good thing. In our culture, "getting a person stirred up" is often seen as negative, and much energy is spent maintaining a facade of politeness, avoiding controversial subjects, keeping up appearances at all costs. This attitude is poisonous in caregiving, especially in being with someone in grief. No one is helped by forced cheerfulness. If anything, an encounter with a caregiver who avoids stirring up anything unpleasant leaves everyone feeling drained and lonely. Allowing difficult things to

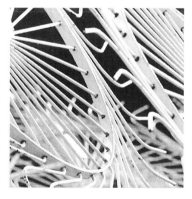

be spoken, even if they bring up old griefs and reopen wounds, creates space in the pain for the healing air of God. Layers of grief under the surface are brought to the light. The breath of the Spirit releases the pain, just as the fierce sun draws out moisture in hay.

Carol Hodgdon, speaking from her farm in Randolph, Vermont, tells me there is a secret to tedding correctly: you can't go fast. If the tractor speed is too great, the hay is flung out in weird directions and the damp underlayers are left on the ground. You have to go slowly. Even so the tedding of our hearts cannot be hastened. We must be patient and gentle as we lift up our own memories, griefs, and struggles to the light. And we must be exceedingly patient and gentle with others. We simply stand with them through their own torturous process and listen. We offer to accompany others at their own pace. We cannot rush them to get over their grief and get on with their life, an often-heard message that leaves them feeling guilty, shamed, and isolated. Tedding of hay and grief, to be complete at all levels, must be done slowly.

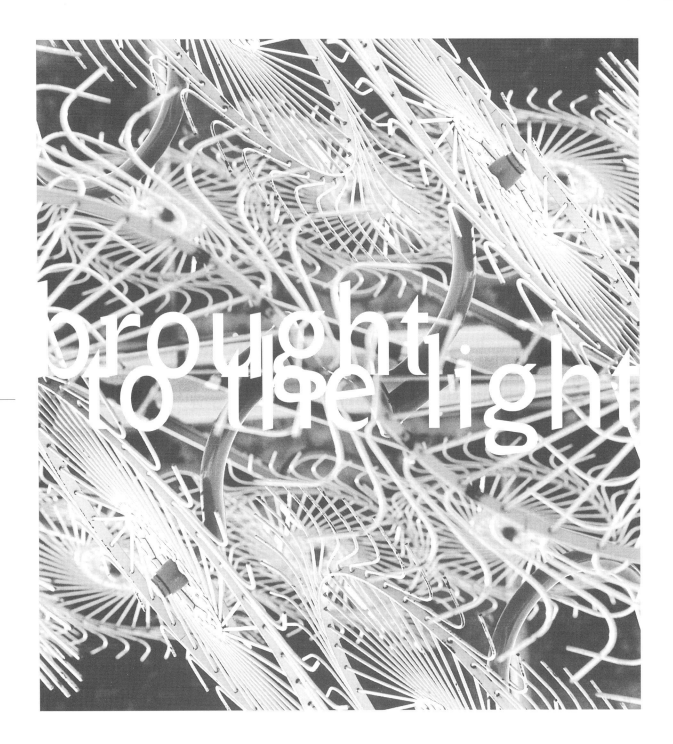

brought to the light

Paul wrote to Timothy, "I am reminded of the sincerity of
your faith, a faith which was alive in Lois your grandmother
and Eunice your mother before you, and which, I am
confident, lives in you also. That is why I now
remind you to stir into flame the gift of God
which is within you" (2 Timothy 1:5–6
NEB). Paul's words teach us that God's
presence is already here, already within
us, to heal and bless. As hearts are
stirred, the gift of God is rekindled—heat
and light within. The tedding wheels
turn, old sorrows are brought to light, and
in the fragrant summer air all is made well.

Make "little Sabbaths."

Pause often for a breath of renewal during the day.

X out some time on your calendar to remain empty this week
and next.

X is the symbol for Christ.

You are Christ-ing the time.

X is a kiss.

You are opening up a time to be kissed by the Spirit.

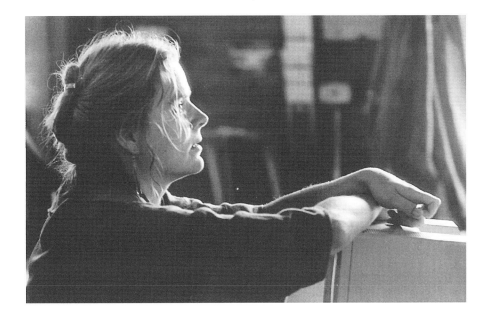

"little Sabbaths"

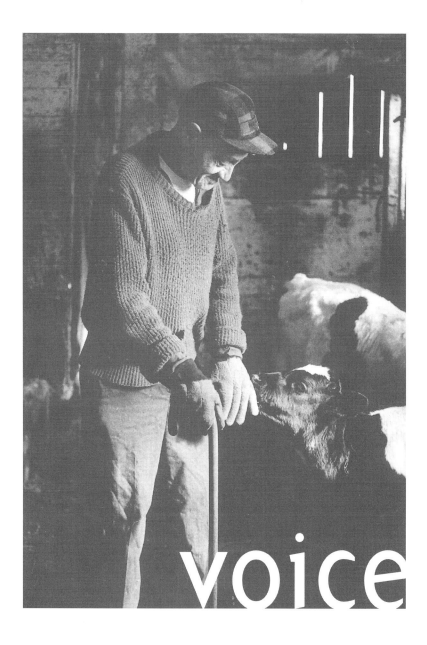

voice

This can be sung unaccompanied or with a simple improvised arrangement
on available instruments. Cello solo on the melody is particularly
effective.

I Heard the Voice of Jesus Say

Words: Horatius Bonar, 1846, alt.

Music: Kathy Wonson Eddy, 1983

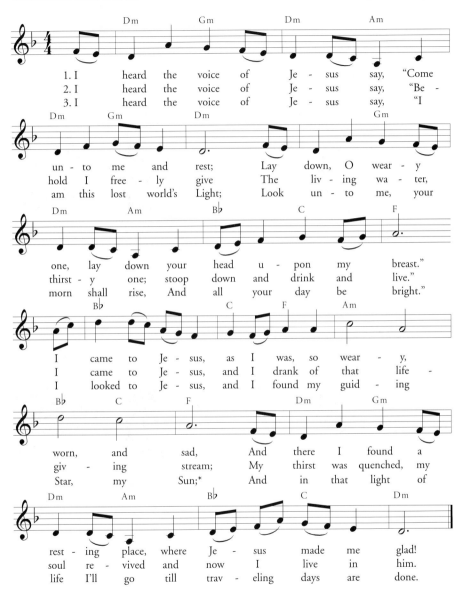

1. I heard the voice of Je - sus say, "Come un - to me and rest; Lay down, O wear - y one, lay down your head u - pon my breast." I came to Je - sus, as I was, so wear - y, worn, and sad, And there I found a rest - ing place, where Je - sus made me glad!

2. I heard the voice of Je - sus say, "Be - hold I free - ly give The liv - ing wa - ter, thirst - y one; stoop down and drink and live." I came to Je - sus, and I drank of that life - giv - ing stream; My thirst was quenched, my soul re - vived and now I live in him.

3. I heard the voice of Je - sus say, "I am this lost world's Light; Look un - to me, your morn shall rise, And all your day be bright." I looked to Je - sus, and I found my guid - ing Star, my Sun;* And in that light of life I'll go till trav - eling days are done.

75

* On the word "sun" in verse three, D major can be played instead of F and the word held.

I love this photograph because the chairs are empty. The chairs remind me that as a caregiver, sometimes the best thing I can offer is a ministry of absence. There are times when the most loving gift I can give is to allow people the space to experience their pain, sort through their feelings, work out their own solutions. They discover in the process their own capability and God's ever-present love. In our service to others we can confuse caregiving with rushing in to fix, prevent, or solve, as if everything depended on us alone. We can grow into the habit of offering others distraction or anesthesia for their pain. We can become compulsive in our service, never feeling we have done enough. Our ministry of absence can teach us how much we have come to depend on our helpfulness to others for our own self-image. In stepping back from the obsessive giving of care, we can find once more that we are fundamentally cherished children of God, beloved not for what we do, but simply for who we are. An empty chair is a great place to learn this.

My grandmother used to say a chair beckoned her every afternoon to leave her tasks and come "invite her soul," letting the rest of the world take care of itself for a while. Her phrase "invite my soul" is just right; it speaks of the truth that in emptiness and silence we find abundance. In solitude there is actually deep companionship. The visitor we invite to sit with us is our very soul, a lively friend indeed, a wise teacher and imaginative child.

These three chairs are waiting. They manifest an openness to whatever lies ahead. Their arms are outstretched to harsh winds and bitter cold. Yet the chairs seem to say, "We will wait this out. Summer's joys and relaxation will come again." The passage of winter to spring happens in miniature within us whenever we sit in stillness in an empty chair and "invite our soul." At first we may become more aware of pain in the present, harsh and bitter realities we have been denying in our busy conscious life. However, as we sit, we come to know strength and hope. We become more and more certain of summer and rebirth and warmth to come. The people we love, from whom we are absent as we enjoy this empty time, are enriched by our "soul's visit" when we return to them.

The word "empty" is from the Indo-European root *med,* which also gives us the English words "medicine," "remedy," and "meditation." It is fascinating that in the very

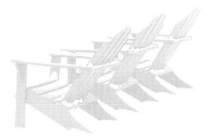

The visitor we invite to sit with us is our very soul, a lively friend indeed, a wise teacher and imaginative child.

roots of our language emptiness is connected not only with meditation (to think things over, to reflect), but also with agents of healing, with medicinal, curative power. The ancients knew a deep truth we need to relearn in our busy culture. Our own healing is found in the empty chair where we invite our soul and open ourselves to whatever the future brings. Our soul, *anima,* brings healing in her gentle hands from the Great Physician. Emptiness offers holy medicine to refresh and inspire.

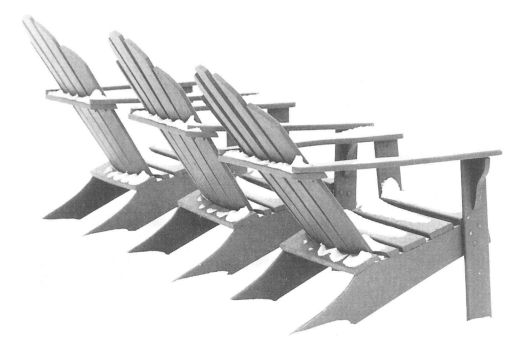

"invite our soul"

it speaks of the truth that in
emptiness and silence we find
abundance.
In solitude there is actually
deep companionship.

imitators

Therefore be imitators of God,

as beloved children,

and live in love,

as Christ loved us.

—Ephesians 5:1

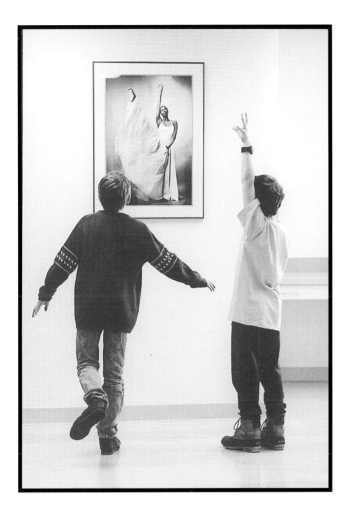

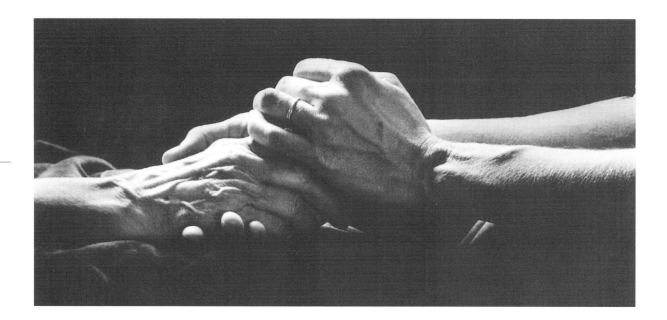

Ten days before his death Rabbi Abraham Heschel had taped a television interview for NBC. At the close of the program the interviewer asked him if he had a special message for young people. He nodded his head and seemed to turn to the future he would never see. "Remember," he said, "that there is meaning beyond absurdity. Know that every deed counts, that every word is power. . . . Above all, remember that you must build your life as if it were a work of art."

every deed counts
every word is power

every word is power

Abraham Joshua Heschel, *I Asked for Wonder: A Spiritual Anthology,* edited with introduction by Samuel H. Dresner (New York: Crossroad, 1985), viii-ix. © 1985 by the Crossroad Publishing Company. Used by permission of the Crossroad Publishing Company.

Every person has a priceless treasure to offer others:
full attentiveness.
Your whole, undivided attention,
given to another,
is of inestimable value,
a luminous gift.

Today,
practice attentiveness.

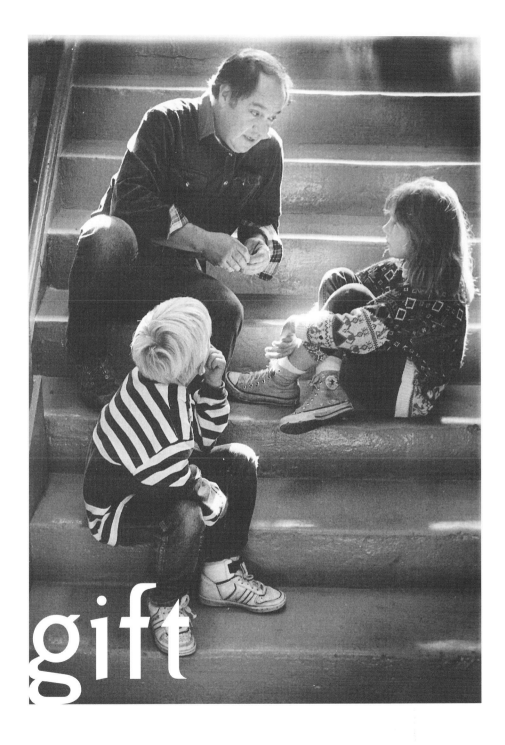

gift

For a long time I have made a
spiritual practice of writing in my
journal early each day. Before first
light I go to my sermon desk and
allow stream-of-consciousness writing to
flow. These pages become daily letters to
God, sharing my thanksgiving for the little
gifts of the previous day and my need for God's
help in the day that stretches before me. As I
write, the sun rises over the ridge of mountains to
the east of our home and the light pours over my
hands and onto the page. Slanted yellow light pools on
my desk and blazes, coppery, on the edges of branches outside the window. Here are words that emerged during one
January sunrise:

K: What is your word for me today, God?

GOD: Blessing. "I will bless you, that you will be a bless-
        ing" (Genesis 12:2).

        Look closely: Blessing. LESS is in there! Less effort-ful
        life; instead, ease. Less future-orientation; instead,
        mindfulness in the present.

        Look closely: Blessing. SING is in there! Sing my praise!
        My song is in your life this day. Let all you do today
        be a song. All you do!

        Look closely: What is left? Just the letter *B*. JUST BE!
        That is all. That is enough.

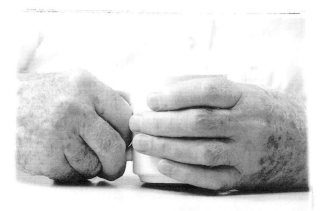

blessing

In 1983 our family lived in Wales for a five-month sabbatical study of Celtic Christianity. We discovered that for early Celtic Christians, blessing was a critical element in everyday life. There were special blessings for each daily act: lighting the peat fire, clothing the body, washing the children, planting, walking a path to a neighbor's home, weaving, fishing, going to sleep—a prayer for God's blessing accompanied every action. Irish scribes would put the mark Xb at the top of each new page of calligraphy or illuminated manuscript. This sign, meaning "Christe benedicte," was a prayer for Christ to bless that day's work. Each stroke of the pen was thus blessed by God. May you live each day under the sign Xb, the benediction of Christ on all you do. May the blessing of LESS, of SINGing, of JUST BE-ing grow in you like the clear light of a January sunrise.

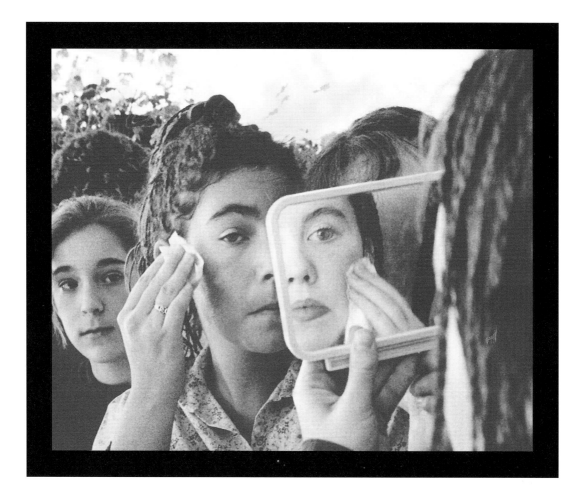

This is very beautiful when signed using hand motions that express the
words. It can be sung unaccompanied, or with an improvised piano
accompaniment and violin, horn, flute, and two voices.

Bless, O Christ, My Face

Words: Celtic prayer

Music: Kathy Wonson Eddy, 1996

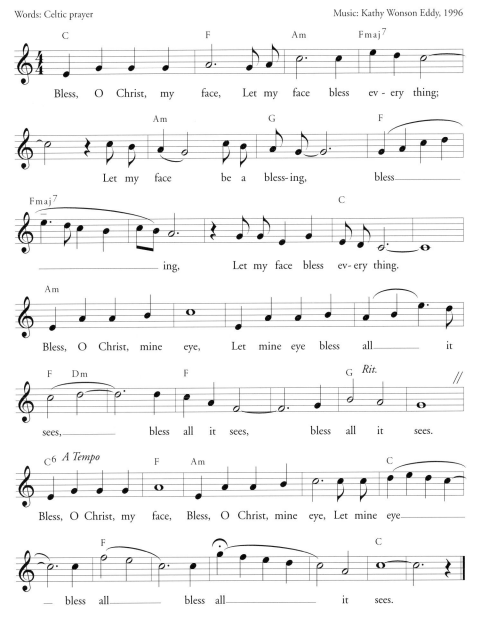

Words: Prayer by Mary MacLeod, Naast, Gairloch, as quoted in *Carmina Gadeliea*, vol. 3, ed. Alexander Carmichael (Edinburgh, Scotland: The Scottish Academic Press). © The Scottish Academic Press. Used by permission. Tune: Copyright © 1996 Kathy Wonson Eddy.

Let the light of late afternoon
shine through chinks in the barn, moving
up the bales as the sun moves down.

Let the cricket take up chafing
as a woman takes up her needles
and her yarn. Let evening come.

Let dew collect on the hoe abandoned
in long grass. Let the stars appear
and the moon disclose her silver horn.

Let the fox go back to its sandy den.
Let the wind die down. Let the shed
go black inside. Let evening come.

To the bottle in the ditch, to the scoop
in the oats, to air in the lung
let evening come.

Let it come, as it will, and don't
be afraid. God does not leave us
comfortless, so let evening come.

—*Jane Kenyon*

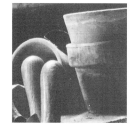

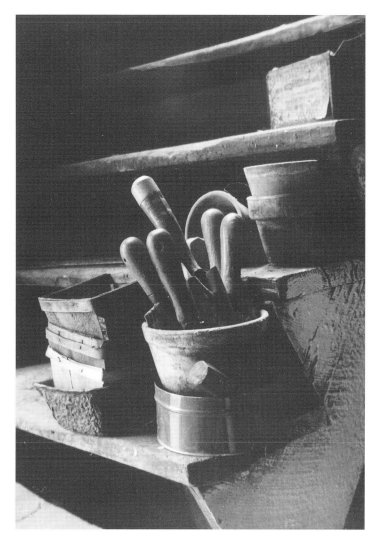

Let the stars

appear and

the moon

disclose her

silver horn.

power
and grace

Once when Bob and I went on retreat to Weston Priory, the text for the day was the visitation of Mary to Elizabeth (Luke 2:39–56). One of the brothers spoke with feeling during the silent reflection after the scripture was read. He said he had a picture in his mind of Elizabeth stretching out her hands toward Mary's belly, and he had come to know that gesture as a call for each of us. He said we are each invited to witness the way God is being born in others' lives and to speak of it. We are to say, "I behold God in you. . . . I see how God is coming to birth in your life." It is a gift of power and grace when we offer this witness, for it reminds others that they are vessels of God and God is at work in them.

Childbirths are never easy and rarely timely. Mary's pregnancy as an unwed teenager was certainly not at a convenient time. Spiritual births are difficult as well: the birthing of a new depth of commitment, or love, or self-understanding is a painful process. When we say, "I see God in you in this process; God is bringing something to birth in your life," we are giving courage for the arduous labor ahead. We are sharing our awe at life, at the boundless creativity of God to bring the new into being.

The brother at Weston closed his meditation by looking out at the congregation intently. He said, "We are each pregnant. God is in us. God is being born in new ways in our lives. I see God in you." And he stretched forth his hands.

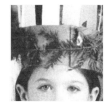

We carry light within us.

There is no need merely to reflect.

Others carry light within them.

These lights must wake to each other.

—M. C. Richards

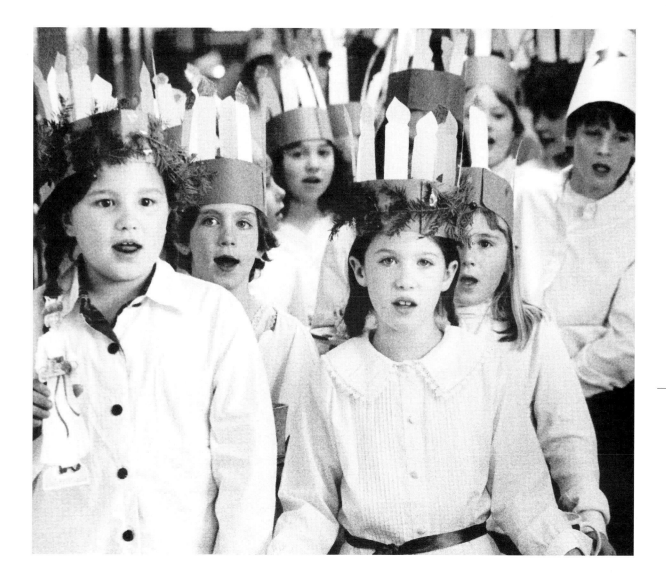

M. C. Richards, *Centering in Poetry, Pottery, and the Person,* 2nd ed.
(Hanover, N.H.: Wesleyan University Press, 1989), 18. © 1989 by
Mary Caroline Richards. Used by permission of the University Press
of New England.

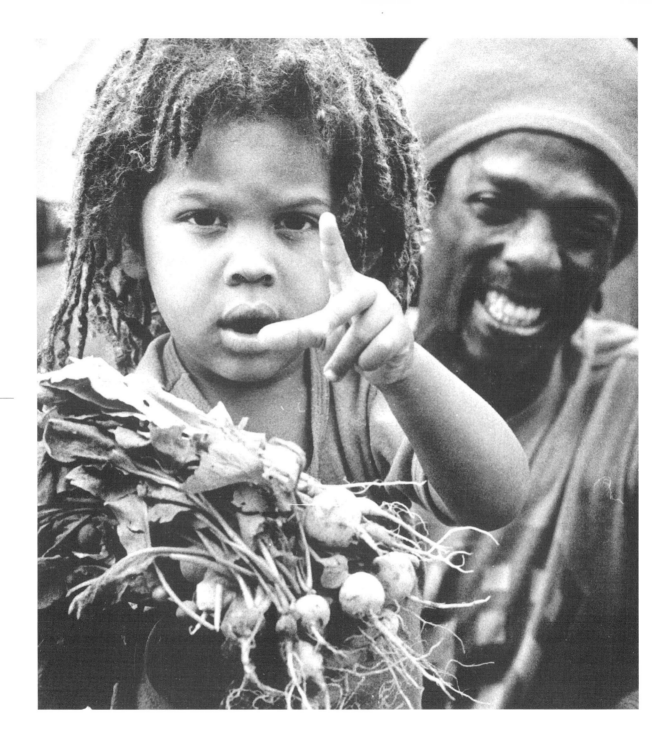

all creation

For the Fruit of All Creation

Words: F. Pratt Green, 1970

Music: Kathy Wonson Eddy, 1990

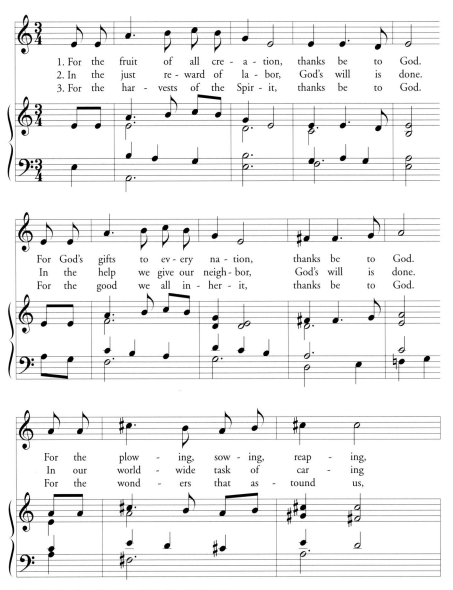

1. For the fruit of all cre-a-tion, thanks be to God.
2. In the just re-ward of la-bor, God's will is done.
3. For the har-vests of the Spir-it, thanks be to God.

For God's gifts to ev-ery na-tion, thanks be to God.
In the help we give our neigh-bor, God's will is done.
For the good we all in-her-it, thanks be to God.

For the plow-ing, sow-ing, reap-ing,
In our world-wide task of car-ing
For the wond-ers that as-tound us,

98

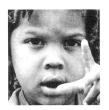

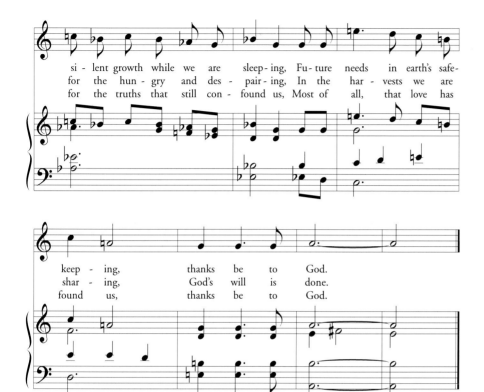

si - lent growth while we are sleep-ing, Fu-ture needs in earth's safe-
for the hun-gry and des-pair-ing, In the har-vests we are
for the truths that still con - found us, Most of all, that love has

keep - ing, thanks be to God.
shar - ing, God's will is done.
found us, thanks be to God.

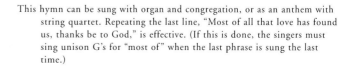

This hymn can be sung with organ and congregation, or as an anthem with string quartet. Repeating the last line, "Most of all that love has found us, thanks be to God," is effective. (If this is done, the singers must sing unison G's for "most of" when the last phrase is sung the last time.)

All things of the earth
Sing of God.

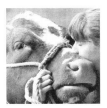

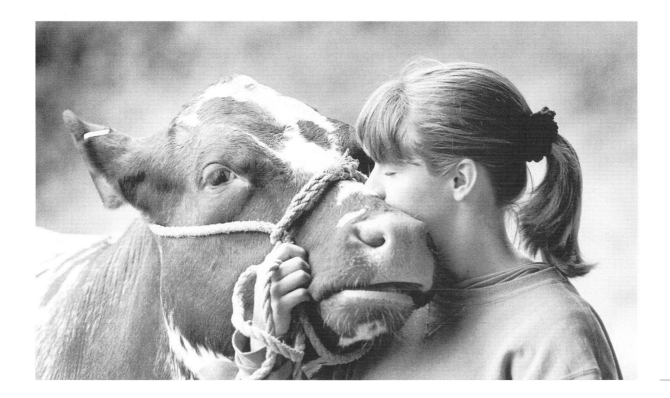

All photographs were taken with Nikon 35mm equipment and Kodak T-MAX film unless otherwise noted.

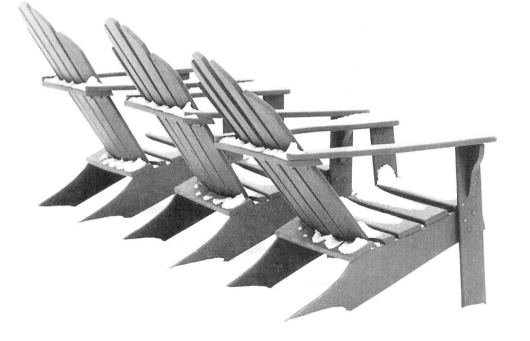

List of Photographs

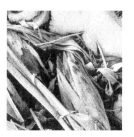

pages 4, 103 *November Corn*

Pinello cornfield, Randolph Center, Vermont.

pages 6, 7 *Shakari*

Senior at Dartmouth College. Photographed for
Dartmouth 1994 annual report.

page 8 *The Kiss*

The birthing center of Gifford Medical Center,
Randolph, Vermont.

pages 10, 104 *The Orb Weaver*

Peter Wakefield at the West Brookfield Community
Church, West Brookfield, Vermont.

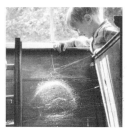

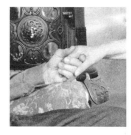

page 13 *Eucharist at the Senior Center*

At the annual Thanksgiving meal at Randolph Senior
Citizen Center, cranberry sauce is passed among
friends.

pages 15, 16, 17 *Dove at the Window*

A transparent printed dove hung at our kitchen window for many years. One winter day the late-afternoon
sun created this image.

page 18 *Street Sweeper*

Randolph suffered three devastating fires in its small
downtown district within one year. This boy joined in
community clean-up efforts.

page 21 *Advent 1989*

Christ Episcopal Church, Bethel Gilead, Vermont.

pages 22, 23, 104 *Vermont Couple*

I'd been sent to East Randolph to photograph this
couple. After forty-five minutes of conversation and a

tour of the dirt-floored cellar where keg cider and hundreds of mason jars stored the previous summer's harvest, this photograph was taken. I left with a jar of the best dill pickles I've ever tasted.

page 24 *Didgeridoo*

Photographed at the New World Festival of Celtic and French Canadian Music, Labor Day weekend, Randolph, Vermont. Why aboriginal instruments from Australia were being sold I'm not sure, but I'm glad they were.

pages 26, 27 *Florence Scholl Cushman*

Florence Scholl Cushman's piano studio, Randolph, Vermont.

pages 28, 31 *Three Trees*

Photographed while lying on my back in a rain-filled cart path on Good Friday (Kodak Tri X).

page 32 *Freezing and Thawing*

Sometimes high humidity and rapidly dropping temperatures conspire to create ice with no storm. Such was the case at a magical spot between 1,200 and 1,300 feet as I descended from our home on Braintree Ridge down into Randolph Village.

pages 34, 35, 37, 105 *Dundee Voices of Joy*

Singers from Dundee South Africa on the stage of Chandler Music Hall, Randolph, Vermont, June 1995 (Kodak TMZ).

page 38 *Stage Whisper*

Spring dance recital, Chandler Music Hall, Randolph, Vermont (Kodak TMZ).

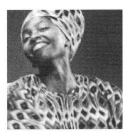

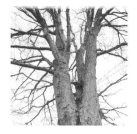

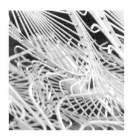

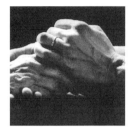

pages 60, 63 *Mud Season*

    If you want to visit Vermont friends in the spring, you'd be wise to call first!

page 65 *Sledding*

    Braintree School recess offers an opportunity not found in many elementary schools. Snow began falling heavily just as children started going inside.

page 66 *Simo*

    Photographed at the parsonage after lemonade and conversation as evening fell.

pages 69, 70, 107 *Hay Tedders*

    The back way to Randolph from the Tunbridge World's Fair brings you past agricultural equipment in East Randolph. These hay tedders reminded me of the carnival rides I had just photographed at the fair.

page 73 *The Writer*

    Robin was a colleague of mine at the *Herald of Randolph.* I recorded this moment on the end of an exposed news roll just before disappearing into the darkroom to develop the film.

page 74 *Calf Barn*

    Leon worked with cows all his life. This photograph was taken when the herd was sold.

page 81 *Imitators: The Dance*

    Photographed in a hallway at Gifford Medical Center, Randolph, Vermont.

pages 82, 107 *Hospice*

    Kathy and Helen: the ebb and flow of caregiving.

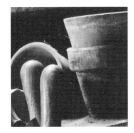

List of Music